LOSING MOTHER TWICE

LOSING MOTHER TWICE

FACING THE ALZHEIMER'S JOURNEY

Life is hard
God is good!
Let's write about it!

Regina Olson and Deborah Harwood

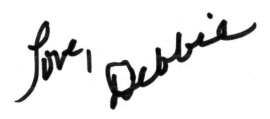

Love, Debbie

The authors of this book do not offer professional medical advice to individual readers. The views expressed are the perspective of the authors. Ideas and suggestions presented herein are not intended as a substitute for consultation with a qualified physician.

The list of references consulted in the writing of this book are provided to help readers explore information and research regarding Alzheimer's disease, dementia, health, and nutrition. The authors have attempted to cite documentation in accessible sources. Some web addresses and links may have changed since publication.

ISBN-13: 9781539516057
ISBN-10: 1539516059
Library Of Congress Control Numbers: 2016917211
CreateSpace Independent Publishing Platform
North Charleston, South Carolina

For Blake, Audrey, Alice, Noah, Max, Taylor, and Abigail

TABLE OF CONTENTS

INTRODUCTION

We lost Mother to Alzheimer's disease almost 10 years before we lost her to death. Our story tells of Mother's progressive decline as she struggled with the disease that took her from us . . . even while her physical body survived . . . even though she no longer knew who we were . . . even when she could no longer say, "I'm ready. I don't know why the good Lord doesn't take me."

For those who also watch aging parents, failing spouses, or declining siblings struggle with dementia, we know how incredibly difficult it is to watch a loved one lose herself. Our story may be your story as well.

My sister Debbie and I began writing about Mother's illness as emotional therapy for ourselves—an attempt to make sense of things. The book grew from Debbie's journaling and my essay in 2007 for the Alzheimer's Foundation of America magazine, *AFA Care Quarterly*. Writing that essay, which later became the first chapter of *Losing Mother Twice,* helped me grasp the nature of the impending sojourn that awaited our mother.

We continued to write as our family watched her navigate the treacherous path of the Alzheimer's journey. It was a journey set in place by the tangles and plaques in her brain, and it lasted until she could no longer find her way through the brambled path.

What we learned about facing Alzheimer's disease is clear to us now. Clarity was not so easy to achieve when we were in the middle of it . . . while our mother was leaving us in slow motion. In the thick of it, we realized we were not very good at handling the difficulties of a parent whose memory was skipping out before the end of her ride. We were better with problems we could fix with duct tape and determination.

For this challenge we needed to know facts about the disease we were up against. We dug into Alzheimer's research, much of which is complex and all of which has yet to offer definitive data as to causes and cures. We had dozens of questions. We wanted to understand, for example, the difference between Alzheimer's disease and other forms of dementia. We wanted to find out why Mother remembered the words to her favorite old hymns but could not remember our names. Finding answers to many of our questions, we continued to write. Consequently, while our story chiefly relates what we discovered while facing our mother's condition, it also offers a survey of the research that helped us understand the nature of the disease that was taking her.

We have attempted to make complex information understandable by placing it within the context of our mother's life—one person among the millions afflicted by the common tragedy that is Alzheimer's disease. She was our sampling size of one, a real person with a family who loved her, separated affectionately from the statistical norm.

Please note that we have decided to tell the story in one voice. A clearer story emerges when the narrator speaks using "I" to relay the experience of either of the authors. Our goal is to convey what is true or, at least, what is true as we see it. Most of what we understand about losing our mother to Alzheimer's disease we know only by looking back.

Regina Wood Olson

CHAPTER 1
FAULTLESS

> To be fully alive, fully human,
> and completely awake
> is to be continually thrown from the nest.
> ~ PEMA CHODRON

Six cans of Faultless spray starch in Mother's laundry room brought me to tears as I sat cross-legged on the floor, counting can after can. Mother must have been buying another each time she went grocery shopping. I clutched one of the white aerosol cans, studying its blue lettering and red star. I stared at others around the room: an empty can on the dryer, a partially used one on the shelf with the iron, two stored on the water softener, and one by the hamper. How curious. Six cans of spray starch would force me to face the reality of Mother's condition.

I recalled the strange e-mail my sister had sent me after she had visited Mom to help her with cleaning tasks Mother could no longer accomplish. Debbie counted nine banana peels and thirteen empty yogurt containers under Mother's bed. I understood her numerical survey of the damage only after I found myself counting cans of starch. The progression of Alzheimer's disease was calculable.

Mother, of course, could not be blamed for something so silly as having too much spray starch on hand. She couldn't remember. This failure of memory, her constant repeating of stories, her forgetting answers to questions she had asked moments before—all of these were lapses our family had rationalized away. Perhaps we hoped she would snap out of it.

While I was still on the floor, Mother appeared at the doorway. "Just put that starch in here," she said, pointing to a laundry basket. "I'll get to the ironing tomorrow." But by tomorrow, she would have forgotten about the basket of clothes to be ironed.

I remember my mother ironing when I was young—usually Tuesdays, just as her embroidered dish towels directed. Such pride she took in stiff white pinafores over blue gingham dresses for her girls. In the days before permanent press, she ironed handkerchiefs, pillowcases, and underwear. A clean house and neatly dressed children were signs of her worth. It explained why she didn't want anyone showing up to clean her bedroom or reorganize the laundry room.

Pulling myself off the floor with spray starch in hand, I grabbed the ironing board and began to work on the basket of clothes. I am my mother's daughter, after all, and needed to accomplish something—anything—to forestall thinking about what the spray starch and banana peels and yogurt containers meant.

My thoughts drifted to the past. When I was a child, Mother sometimes sprinkled clothes with water, rolled them up, and stored them in the freezer for ironing after other chores were done. I tried to recall how she soaked the wash in a thickened starch solution—maybe it was called bluing, or perhaps that was for whitening clothes. I don't recall now. It was so long ago. My urge was to ask her, but that would have put her on the spot. And I had not yet negotiated the delicate balance between exercising memory's neural pathways and embarrassing her with requests for information she could not supply. So many memories had slipped away. No chance of her now recalling what she had eaten for breakfast.

At this early point in the disease, the family deferred the future with humor. Before we knew what was wrong with Mother, we joked that the good thing about Alzheimer's was you were always meeting new people and you could hide your own Easter eggs. Very little humor in that now. My sisters and I worked at stopgap measures: using a timed medicine dispenser, arranging who would hear what the doctor said, taking the car keys, reminding her to bathe. To avoid her resistance to being managed, we developed the strategy of blaming whichever sibling was not present at the time. The problem of caring for an aging parent seemed easier when I read about it in books and magazines because, of course, the experience was happening to someone else.

No longer able to hold back the tears, I stepped outside into the cool night to look at the stars. I searched the sky. So many stars, a sliver of a moon. I wondered about stars and heredity and who was at fault.

As I was growing up, Mom had often shared the story about how I had cried for the moon and the stars when a very young child and how my grandfather said he would get them for me. "We'll get you that star!" my grandfather promised. When telling me the story, Mother always quoted his exact words, but she feigned displeasure. I imagined her scolding her father-in-law for spoiling her child. I also thought about how Mother was so like the stars she could no longer name. The light still traveled through the universe, though the star itself was long since gone.

The chill in the air forced me inside. I picked up the can of spray starch, having work to finish and having found no one to blame.

CHAPTER 2

FIRST SIGNS

> If you're riding ahead of the
> herd, take a look back
> every now and then to make sure it's still there.
> ~ WILL ROGERS

The family watched Mother's illness advance, surprised and alarmed by each new event that revealed change and loss. After the doctor used the words "Alzheimer's disease," we found something to blame for the dramatic changes in Mother's cognitive abilities and our own confusing pile of emotions. Having a diagnosis—or as much of a diagnosis as anyone received at that time . . . there had been a series of cognitive tests—didn't change anything for Mother. The doctor had downplayed the significance of the disease, saying most people fall, break a hip, and die of complications before they die of Alzheimer's disease. We were alarmed but not surprised by the diagnosis, which explained everything about Mom's behavior. It voiced everything we had not been able to say, and it made us recognize that Mother's losses had started earlier than we had been willing to admit.

We think this is true for most families facing the problem of a parent's decline. The little failures in memory, the moments of confusion, the repetitions—all slip by, unacknowledged.

Mother was skillful in covering up and quick to defend herself. We backed down and backed off. Confronting our intelligent and capable mother by noting her mental lapses felt like a betrayal of some unspoken rule of allegiance.

We suppose the first point at which most families deal with Alzheimer's disease is when the loved one starts getting lost . . . when they are unable to find their way home. Being at home and being forgetful is different from being missing. Mother's youngest granddaughter, Katie, was the first to say the words: "Grandma got lost!" The six-year-old child whispered the truth like revealing a secret, her chubby fingers cupped to the side of her mouth as she emphasized the words to her mother, my sister Lori. Grandma had driven Katie home, and they took almost an hour to make the ten-minute trip.

Some weeks later, in a phone conversation, Mother told me about a second experience, almost as an afterthought in the conversation. She had gotten lost while driving home from church. Mom was nonchalant, her demeanor equivalent to her having said she had misplaced her keys that morning.

"I haven't told anyone," she said. But I already knew. Lori had called to tell me about this second time Mom had gotten lost. My first thought when I found out she had driven around the Indiana countryside while looking for something familiar, some marker to identify the way home, was "Thank God for Indiana county roads!" Even numbers run east-west; odd numbers run north-south. Perfect squares. I imagined Mom driving around making left turns until she returned repeatedly to the same place.

At some point, she had driven straight on County Road 21 and ended up at a gas station across from the middle school. She went in to ask for directions. They told her the middle school was across the street, the city park was down the road, and the golf course was the other direction. When they mentioned Greene Road, she knew where she was. At one time, she and

Dad had lived on Greene Road; they had been there for over 20 years. Her two youngest children had gone to the school she had not recognized, but it had then been called a junior high. Perhaps that added to the confusion, we reasoned, even while knowing that between basketball games, other school functions, and picking up and dropping off kids, she had been there hundreds of times. She made it home, two hours later than normal. It was left turn, left turn, left turn until she squared her way home.

It's amazing to us now that no alarm bells started ringing in anyone's head. We simply did nothing. Getting lost happened just those two times—as far as we knew. Everyone gets turned around occasionally. She didn't offer much of an explanation to Dad. She said she had been driving around, which, of course, was true. She didn't want him to know.

But he already knew; he had seen the other signs. We all had. She repeatedly complained the family was withholding information from her. "Why didn't anyone tell me?" was the common accusation, even though she had been told and then told again later.

We did not know yet which details she would retain until the time of the recital or the game or the family gathering. But we knew for sure she would be surprised when it was time to attend those events. Although the episodes of getting lost were most worrisome, repetition of stories, details, and questions was most predominant.

We began calling Mother's repetitions The Story of the Day. With a shrinking number of stories available in her memory, she often relied on visual cues to engage in conversation. For a brief time, she told the story of finding the sapphire ring each time she looked down at her hand. Telling and retelling the story was her contribution to the day's dialogue. The story differed slightly with each telling but always started with a question: "Did I ever tell you where I got this ring?" She had told each of us, often.

Sometimes in the beginning stages of her illness, she could stop herself and say, "I've already told you that haven't I?"

The retelling of a story shapes the past with each telling. We rationalized that this phenomenon is true for all of us. It wasn't just Mom. In retelling, different events are given prominence or an alternate perspective is explored. In the mind of the teller, a story can be reshaped to account for motives in sharing the story and the audience to whom it is told. Telling true history is a tricky business even for someone with a good memory. Everyone knows that if five people retell the same story, five different versions emerge.

We know now that variations in Mother's stories occurred because she was losing chunks of her past. Her mind was supplying probable scenarios to bridge the gaps in memory. We also noticed she became more bold and forthright in her reinvented life. In new versions, she was quick to right wrongs, give inspirational advice, or save situations from near disaster. The events she described filled in what she could not remember. These events might have happened, but did not. Her stories' details shifted; some of her stories were completely false. Hers was a malleable truth—the specific details changing in a pattern that became recognizable.

The family first recognized Mom's habit of changing details in stories one time when several of us returned home for a birthday celebration. She explained and re-explained why her arm was sore. With a slight hint of a Southern accent returning to her speech, she talked about how her young grandson, Ryan, ran through the living room, slipping past her chair. Their playful game included extending her arm to request a toll. We all knew that game. He would make the imaginary payment and duck underneath. As he grew taller, Ryan found it difficult to duck far enough, and one day, he caused her arm to hyperextend. Her arm was sore for several days. Her version of this story changed in the next telling. Another grandson, Jonathan—at that time

22 years old—was the little boy who had run past her chair. Soon after, the story changed again so that the child who caused the injury by failing to duck under her arm was Lori, Ryan's mother. It seemed like a simple case of using the wrong name, but the hard truth was that she was living in the foggy territory of her fading memory and her brain was providing her with no road signs.

We are sure it's true that families retell stories because shared experiences knit them together. Family stories chart their unique experiences—getting caught in the snowstorm in Lake Tahoe, taking the eventful trip to an amusement park, witnessing the near tragedy when the little boy next door found his father's gun and brought it out to play. These stories are shared joys and troubles we never tire of telling precisely because everyone knows how the story ends. It was easy to classify Mom's retelling of events as a part of this familial urge. Looking back, we know her stories were repeated not because we knew them well but because she thought we did not know them at all.

The signs of Alzheimer's disease were right there for us to see.

CHAPTER 3

WATCHING GRANDMA DANCE

At the end of the day, stories
are about what you lose.
~ JOHN IRVING

When the family gathered for my daughter's wedding, all of Mother's daughters—Regina, Pam, Debbie, and Lori—watched her behavior closely. How she managed the wedding would be an important marker in judging the progress of the disease. At the wedding dance, we learned that of all the things Mother lost to the disease, her memory was just one of them.

The evening of the wedding Debbie rose in the middle of the night to write about the day in her journal. She wondered whether or not our mother would remember any of it. She described the beautiful setting, the gorgeous bride—so glowing with happiness, the flowing satin gown that twirled around her as she and the groom danced their first dance. And Grandma, there, dancing too.

Her dancing amazed the family most. We had expected that she would continually ask what we were doing there and who was getting married. She had lost the ability to remember why she was getting dressed up. Since she could no longer complete simple tasks, we had expected that her daughters would need to get her ready for the wedding.

Yet, we had not expected her to dance. She had been raised—and raised her five children—in a church that strictly forbade dancing. The old joke goes that church members frowned on sex standing up because it might lead to dancing. We daughters shared that joke many years past our adolescence and never in the presence of our mother.

Mother had not danced at the weddings of her children in deference to her fundamentalist belief. She had not danced at previous weddings of grandchildren, though she did not object to their wedding dances following the receptions. She did not ridicule or preach. For all of her life, she had accepted the rules presented to her. Perhaps Mother enjoyed seeing her family celebrate, but she was too schooled in proper conduct to dance at those previous weddings—too uncomfortable, too ready to avoid any display of effervescent behavior, too reticent to call attention to herself.

This wedding of a granddaughter was different. At the urging of my sister, Pam, and because she had lost memories of social prescriptions of the past, she consented to be led to the dance floor. She danced in a circle with her family, who held hands and raised them to the beat of the music. She danced with her grandsons. She danced with newlyweds. She danced beyond her presumed limits of endurance, bad knees and all.

At this stage of her disease, Mother was losing memories of her childhood. Long ago, many details of her life and the rearing of her children had slipped away. She had lost some aspects of her personality. However, on this day, we knew she had also lost her ability to censor herself, to confine herself to social parameters. On this day, Mother still knew us, and we found joy in what she had lost.

In her journal, Debbie expressed her amazement. "I hope when I am my mother's age," she wrote, "I have lost my mind enough to dance with abandon at my granddaughter's wedding."

CHAPTER 4

FRUSTRATION

> I always like to look on the
> optimistic side of life,
> but I am realistic enough to know
> that life is a complex matter.
> ~ WALT DISNEY

As family members adjusted to our changing relationship with our mother, we were action oriented. Strength was summoned; decisions were made. And we could handle anything—in the short run. The long, mind-numbing dailiness of losing Mom to Alzheimer's, however, required another skill: patience. How could we deal with the frustrations of even the little things? She failed to recall information she had stated moments ago, and no matter how many times we answered her questions, she couldn't recall the answers we provided. Her repetitious questioning was far more exasperating than a child's endless, "Why?"

I turned to the experience of rearing children as the template for "raising Grandma." An abundance of patience had been required for that feat, too. I simply needed to apply the same principles.

I recalled my kids playing in the backyard along with all the other kids being raised by the neighborhood. Joyful times, but not without frustrations. In those days, backyard squabbles were mediated, skinned knees were bandaged, and children were chauffeured to piano lessons or sports. I sat through countless sporting events—some of them exciting, some quite agonizing. The earliest games were T-ball.

Five-year-olds playing T-ball presented many frustrations. Any given game might find at least one child sitting crisscross applesauce in the middle of center field as if he were waiting for the librarian to start story time. I would groan from my lawn chair as the ball rolled past him and the coach yelled, "Get up, get up!" Then there was the certainty of little boys scuffling in the dirt about who should play second base. I knew my son Ross would be looking on, wanting to yell in his best umpire voice, "Just play ball!" Some little guy would invariably run to third base instead of first when he by chance hit the ball. But he would learn, just as my children had. They learned the game by playing ball all day in the backyard, playground, or empty lot using whatever was available to serve as the bases. A squished pop can could be first base; the little maple tree, second base; the yellow Frisbee, third. It was in the backyard that my kids learned how to hit the ball, run the bases, move the Frisbee when their sister wasn't looking—the basics. It was a slow process.

I tried to hide my lack of patience. I sat in my lawn chair and cheered them on, all the while fretting over their inability to follow instructions and their snail's pace progress in developing basic skills. My frustrations with the young players were similar to the feelings I had about Mom when I watched her fail to figure out the simplest of tasks or turn the wrong direction on her way to the bathroom in her own house.

The difference is that those five-year-olds did learn to hit the ball and run to first base, they did learn to settle disputes, and they did grow up. That five-year-old son of mine—the one who ran bases in our backyard, swinging around the little second base maple tree and launching himself toward third so many times that it damaged the tree—became an adult. Years later, I heard him graciously answer Grandma's repeated question—the same question five times in five minutes. He patiently answered her each time, "No, Grandma, I'm not married yet."

Back then, I loved the T-ball rule that said everyone could bat and if everyone scored, the team batting had to go to the outfield. Or, if one team was ahead by ten runs, everyone could quit. I wished it was like that with Mom sometimes: Ask the same question ten times and you get to quit and move on to something else. After an hour of T-ball, you are hoping it ends soon. It's hot and you're tired and you have a million things to do at home . . . and it does end, and the kids do move on to Little League and the lives that are waiting for them. It occurred to me that with Mom, there was only one way this was going to stop. I didn't want to face that. The only thing we lost in backyard ball games was second base, the little maple tree so damaged that it didn't survive my children's childhood. It was a good trade.

CHAPTER 5

TIME TRAVELER

> The past beats inside me like a second heart.
> ~ JOHN BANVILLE, *THE SEA*

recall when Mother was startled to learn it was my 60th birthday. How could that be, she wondered, since she imagined she was only 50. What must it feel like to wake in the morning on a day from the past? I could picture Mother waking to plan her day, only to discover she didn't need to make breakfast for five children or hurry to church to put up a new bulletin board. Did her turned-upside-down life sneak up on her? Was she always startled by not being able to remember? She might have stood in front of an open refrigerator wondering why she had opened it. I can guess that she might have begun to introduce her best friend but failed to recall her name.

She probably looked in the mirror and wondered about the suddenness of her gray hair. At some point, she must have faced the fact that she had a problem. Did she feel disconnected from the world she struggled to identify? Perhaps she felt that something was slightly off—the way a straw appears when refracted in water, a shift of a few millimeters. Did she trudge along ignoring her significant problem, keeping it at bay in her failing brain? Or, did moments of lucidity bring panic? Frustration? Sadness? Was she simply bored after a busy life of going and doing? I have wondered how bad off she really was when she first started getting upset with us for reminding her of things, managing her appointments, and surprising her with information she thought she had not been told.

Often, she referred to events that would have better fit the scenario of her life 20 years earlier. Once she was in a panic to get dressed for work, fearing she would be late until I reminded her she no longer went to work and hadn't for many years. Another time, I heard her tell a friend that she hardly ever drove the car anymore. "I run to get groceries every once in a while, but not often," she said. At that time, she had not driven for several years.

Her remarks revealed she was living in the distant past. Trying to figure out the time period in which Mother believed she was living was difficult. For Mother, this strange time travel must have been exhausting. At times, she became upset if someone pointed out she was confused and talking about something that was true in the past but irrelevant to the present. She must have felt as if she were rudely summoned back to her present confusing life.

When Mom and Dad first considered getting a long-term care insurance policy, they had to meet with an insurance representative and take a mental acuity test. I don't recall knowing about the test until she talked about it later, saying she was glad she had passed. She was relieved not to have that "Al-timer's disease." I thought nothing about the remark at the time. Perhaps she was worried about her memory even then. She might have experienced being disembodied from actual present time. Maybe she felt the comfortable reality of another time period, only to experience the sudden jolt of awareness of the present, less comfortable one.

Mother's neighbor told us her husband who, suffering from Alzheimer's disease, once ranted about needing to find his mother. He packed his suitcase and told his wife he was going to stay at his mother's house. His mother had passed 30 years before, but in his mind, the situation was urgent. A time in the distant past was more real to him than the present. His caregiver wife was patient and loving, but she continually had to deal with his need to return to the past. With Mom, it was an occasional trouble our family confronted.

The problem with time travel is that it's just one more thing. If it had been Mom's only problem, we could have figured out a way to deal with it. But the burdens of dealing with a person with Alzheimer's disease are many. They pile up like straw on a camel's back. Some days, the time-travel problem is the last straw.

CHAPTER 6

LOSING COMMUNICATION

The way we communicate with
others and with ourselves
ultimately determines the quality of our lives.
~ ANTHONY ROBBINS

My sister recites aloud her inward dialogue when she is hurried and needs to accomplish multiple tasks. This narration of her life is important to her ability to process information. The family is accustomed to her soundtrack and doesn't mind it because the result is the ability to organize by considering everyone's needs. At family gatherings, she is able to keep track of who is arriving at what time and whether they have eaten; she knows which young children have had naps and which kid needs one; she finds out whether a movie will be suitable for all the little ears as well as interesting for the older ones. We call her the social director—or the bossy one, if we are being unkind. Yet we are grateful that saying things out loud helps her process information.

I started thinking about how Mother's ability to process information began to fall apart. I discovered she could no longer follow the plot of a television show. "Well, this doesn't make any sense," she would say. Sometimes older people don't get pop culture references in TV shows, so some things don't make sense to them. That was not Mom's problem—or not her only problem. Her difficulty was in processing the ideas presented so that she could understand the context and follow the plot. My father-in-law preferred watching *The Lawrence Welk Show* instead of *American Idol* for several reasons associated with the content. Mother, however, didn't know what year it was.

True, her communication ability was slipping away, but it was an inconsistent and random decline. Some days she seemed perfectly fine. We could convince ourselves that nothing was wrong. We did not factor in that we were doing everything we could to put no stress on her, make no demands for mental acuity. Problem solved.

Mother began using a strategy to which many Alzheimer's victims turn: she began writing everything down. It was her attempt to hold onto facts. She kept a notebook close by and covered the refrigerator with sticky notes. If you talked to her about an upcoming event, she usually said, "I'm going to write that down." Seemed like a good plan. Debbie put a whiteboard on the bedroom door to help her keep track of doctor appointments, medications, and events. Mother took little interest in it. Maybe she wanted to be reminded only of interesting things in her life. We didn't know if jotting something down worked only if she initiated it or if she was getting worse. Eventually, the whiteboard and her notes—her visual cues—could not compensate for memory loss. Things written on the whiteboard or on various scraps of paper or in her notebook served no purpose if she couldn't remember to look at them.

Just as we could not stop our children from growing up, we could not stop our mother from sliding down this slippery slope. At that time, we had not yet heard of Aricept or Namenda, so we were trying to fix little things, unaware of the daunting bigger picture. What we knew for sure was that as Mom's communication skills faltered, she began communicating in strange ways. I'm not sure my siblings and I were really trying to help Mom hang onto communication or if, instead, we were trying to help ourselves feel less uncomfortable with the distressing changes we saw. Somewhere floating around in the back of my mind were the irrational words, "This can't be happening to *us*. We've all been good."

When we stopped attempting to control things that we could not control and actually listened to our mom, we realized she wasn't sufficiently communicating at all. Her first lapses in communication were evident when she became bored by conversations on subjects she didn't know. We realized her comments were increasingly clichéd, safe, and rhetorical, never requiring analysis by the listener and never adding depth to the conversation. Her standard exchanges were easily offered and required little. We now know she disengaged because she could not hold up her end of the conversation. She could not process new information quickly enough to join in. We understood, at last, why she just wanted us to go away and leave her alone.

As her skills for processing language continued to decline, she began contributing to conversations by using a standard set of previously practiced expressions and well-worn phrasing that fit—or nearly fit—the context of the conversation. She was using her very own Homeric similes, her own ready-made material for insertion into conversation in keeping with her personal oral tradition. She was forced to offer the things she could remember to say. This allowed her to be a part of the conversation without really being in it.

Soon after, she refused to engage in conversations with people she didn't know. Once when Mom, my sister Pam, and I were at a shopping mall, we ran into someone with whom my sister worked. Pam introduced her friend, and we all decided to have a cup of coffee at a sidewalk café. Mom and I were meeting this woman for the first time, and I suppose just about everybody knows there are certain niceties—certain socially acceptable chatter that people engage in as they join in and support the conversation of two people with an ongoing relationship. One doesn't sit there like a proverbial bump on a log. But Mother did. She engaged in no part of the conversation. At the time, I considered her rude. As we finished our coffee, she finally said, "Isn't it about time we move along?" I didn't know what Pam's friend thought; perhaps she assumed our normally gracious and congenial mother was uninterested . . . or rather dull. We knew that wasn't our mother. Most likely, simple conversation had become too taxing, and her only alternative was feigned boredom.

I knew her skills were getting worse when Mother pretended to remember an issue or person about whom we were talking. Perhaps she did remember. Perhaps she wished she could remember. Perhaps she was covering up because she knew she had a major problem. Often, she changed the subject to something unrelated. And sometimes she just made up stuff.

Later, I thought about her relationships and friendships during this time. I discovered she no longer had many friends—at least not any with whom she was engaging in good brain-stimulating conversations. Truthfully, I knew little about her relationships. She had her church friends and neighbors, but her "girl friends" were not there anymore. I knew something had happened with one of her two best friends—maybe a falling out about which I didn't know details and in which I should not mettle. I've often wondered if the break in their friendship resulted from Mom's changing personality and ways in which her communication was affected by the onset of Alzheimer's disease. I will never know.

Mother's other close friend was in an accident that damaged her brain. Mother missed the relationship the two of them had shared. Her friend was never quite the same, she said. Little did Mother know that within a year or so, she too would struggle with a damaged brain. Years later—at Mom's funeral, in fact—the husband of this best friend told us that Mom had visited her often after the accident. He told us Mom had been there for his wife long after other friends quit coming. Mom graciously engaged in conversations with his wife despite the disruption in her friend's communication skills. As her friend talked, Mom patiently listened to faulty recollections of events, repetition of information, and references to things that hadn't happened. Her husband recalled one visit with Mom when his wife pointed to a picture of mountains and said they had vacationed there the previous week. Her husband said he knew Mom understood this was not true, but he appreciated that she had not challenged her friend or embarrassed them with questions. Mother worked to make those conversations less stressful for her friend. The irony was not lost on us as we listened to his story.

Another factor in her loss of communication with friends resulted from Mom and Dad's move across town to a 55-and-older community at about the same time the symptoms of AD were showing up. I worried that new neighbors, women her age who could have been her friends, may have assumed she was unfriendly. These new people were not going to become her friends at this point in her condition. At times, she was rude or withdrew because she could no longer easily access information locked away in her brain when neighbors asked about her history. Social engagement uses many areas of the brain, and her brain was locking away information and keeping it from her. When neighbors visited, Dad would sometimes answer for her because he knew that she would have trouble answering their questions. This only made her mad at him for butting in when she was trying to build friendships.

We know that Mother was trying to hang onto conversations in which she wanted to participate, but she was unable to hold onto important threads of thought. She was unable to move a conversation along by introducing new ideas and opinions or reacting to the ideas and opinions of others. So she attempted to control whatever she could in a conversation by saying, "I should tell you about the time . . . " and launching into an oft-repeated story that allowed her to interject a monologue she could easily access from memory. If a memory failed to come, she trivialized the subject of discussion with humor that sidetracked the conversation. As a result of being funny, she avoided questions she could not answer. This shows she was not less smart; she had Alzheimer's disease.

Whatever the circumstances that aided and abetted her loss of communication with friends, Mother was no longer experiencing social interaction that was challenging and reciprocal. I can now look back and see this time in her life as the beginning of the isolation that Alzheimer's disease imposes on its victims.

About the time meaningful conversations with friends and neighbors became too difficult, any conversation on the telephone became impossible. We daughters who didn't live near Mom called her often—perhaps not often enough, but enough to stay in touch. The conversations became increasingly difficult as she lost ability to keep track of which child was calling. We were never sure she knew who we were. More and more, she began to say that we had a bad phone connection or that she couldn't hear us. The problem wasn't her ability to hear; she couldn't *understand* what we were saying. My conversations were reduced to giving her the report of how I was doing and how the kids were. I couldn't ask her questions. She couldn't answer them, and trying just made her anxious. My calls were fewer and fewer. I experienced it as another loss of my mother.

Mother's abilities were best suited to a time before constant and immediate communication. She never owned a cell phone. She never learned to check her bank account balance or send a text message to her grandkids. Perhaps she talked on a cell phone a handful of times, but not easily. She couldn't figure out which end was up. She remembered old telephones—phones with cords. As telephone conversations became increasingly difficult, the family realized that she needed that old-style phone, the kind with an earpiece molded especially for hearing someone, a good grip for her hand, and a well-defined mouthpiece she could speak into. Her phone didn't need to multitask.

Whether she withdrew from conversation, diverted attention from it by humor, faked memory of the subject of discussion, or complained about a poor phone connection, Mother was losing communication. As a result, she was fast becoming disconnected from the present.

The drive up Minnesota's North Shore, with the Sawtooth Mountains to the left and Lake Superior to the right, is a winding journey resplendent with nature's beauty. Tourists make that journey primarily in the fall, when the forested landscape of cool summer yields to an even cooler, more colorful autumn— breathtaking no matter the season. If adventurous travelers take the Gunflint Trail at Grand Marais, they can travel into the pristine Boundary Waters Canoe Area. This wilderness stretches beyond the noise of everyday life, beyond the reach of radio stations, beyond cell phone signal, beyond contact with the rest of the world.

The chance of escaping civilization and its incessant need for communication always thrilled me. That was before Mother began slipping away beyond her brain's ability to receive the signals required to prompt normal communication. We could no longer argue a point of scripture or speculate on the Chicago Cub's chances of getting to the World Series or discuss her plan for the flower garden in the spring. We entered every conversation with the knowledge that at any point she might be "out of the signal's range." When people talk on a cell phone while traveling, knowing that signal loss is coming up ahead, we usually share that expected interruption in communication with the listener: "I'm going to lose you in a few minutes, so I'll call back when I have a signal." But when neural synapses of your mother's brain are conspiring against her, how do you tell her, "I'm going to lose you after a few sentences, Mom, and you may not remember because you will be out of your range of communication. It will be OK until next time, when I will tell you again."

So you don't. You say, "It's OK, Mom."

CHAPTER 7

THE PAIN OF LITTLE THINGS

Some of us think holding on makes us strong,
but sometimes it's letting go.
~ HERMAN HESSE

Everyone in the family was on the lookout for Mother's mental lapses. We evidently needed to chart her decline in areas of her life other than communication. We needed to figure out how bad things were getting. Little losses in ability seemed more jarring at the beginning. The first losses seemed significant because we were newly experiencing them. Later, more tragic failures of mental ability didn't disturb us less, but they were less shocking. The family was vigilant in observing and reporting Mom's behavior.

I remember learning that Mother could no longer negotiate a process of more than three steps. She struggled to assemble a ham, cheese, and lettuce sandwich and stood staring blankly down at it. I was babbling about something I assumed she was still able to find interesting. I walked over to the counter and cut her sandwich in two. An automatic response—filling in the next step—as a parent would reach over and cut up something on a child's plate. She walked away with the sandwich, leaving the bread bag open and the butter knife in the mayonnaise jar. It was such a little thing, but so unlike Mom not to clean up after herself. What concerned me most was her getting stuck on the last step in the process. For every family member a different unsettling little thing revealed the fact of her condition.

My daughter discovered that Grandma was no longer functioning well when she helped her make corn casserole for Thanksgiving dinner. For years Ellen had laughed about how she had helped me in the kitchen when she was a child. She learned years later that no one needs to stir flour, salt, and baking powder as long as I required. I was keeping her busy; she felt she was being a good helper. The time her grandmother became confused and frustrated with the process of making the casserole, she realized she needed to take over. She needed to let her grandmother stir flour. It was a hard thing. The lesson the women of our family took from hearing my daughter relate this story was twofold. First was the realization that Grandma could no longer perform multiple-step tasks; and second, we must face the fact that every time the role reversal happened, we needed to acknowledge pain but move on to the requirements of the moment. People were expecting a corn casserole on the Thanksgiving table. I'm pretty sure Mom was thinking if she put on an apron and everyone else got out of the kitchen, everything would be OK.

Another painful recognition of Mom's condition came for my sister, Pam, when she took Mom to a family reunion. She discovered Mom was more concerned about the past than about the present. Pam had taken photos of her grandkids—Mom's great grandchildren. As she showed Mom an album of pictures, Mom glanced at the photos briefly with not the least bit of interest. Instead, she started a conversation with an elderly aunt in the room. Pam doubted Mom would remember to ask to see the photos later. When Mom pushed the photos aside, she knew Mom had no intention of seeing them. How could a great grandma resist Alex's smile and chubby cheeks or Cassidy's I-can-do-anything stance?

After a while, she again put the pictures in front of Mom, and again she put them aside. Pictures of the present were not why they had come to the family reunion, Pam reasoned. She also realized that Mom had stopped asking about her sons, Mike, Jeff, and Jason—or any children of the other siblings who did not live close to her. Mom was losing memory of them and the idea that there were people out there she was supposed to love. Later in the day, Pam picked up the pictures and put them away, sorrowful that Mom no longer felt joy in seeing her great grandchildren.

CHAPTER 8

THE DOPPELGÄNGER

Being deeply loved by someone
gives you strength,
while loving someone deeply gives you courage.
~ Lao Tzu

At some point, each member of our family realized there was another woman in our mother's body. I didn't know this new woman, and I was not sure I cared to know her. She was not my mom—not *our* mom. The difference between her former self—neat, clean, well mannered—and her disheveled and tactless replacement was shocking.

She became embarrassingly rude. Her social skills were never questioned before the doppelgänger slipped in and our real mother fled. Mother had been a proper Southern lady, extremely mindful of appearances—what the neighbors would think and how her children would reflect her image. Even when she criticized others, she cloaked it in kindness. ("She has her hands full with that third son, bless her heart.") My new mom directly confronted people with questions such as "Are you pregnant or just fat?" Her remarks made me gasp, and I corrected her as if she were a first grader. "Well, all these girls around here could stand to lose a little weight," was her speedy reply.

Sometimes her tactless behavior was simply a cover. Mother's biting comments about being rushed or her glare at a waitress asking for her order were the result of too much stimulation. She could not unscramble information from several people talking at one time or numerous choices on a menu. Unable to do more than one thing at a time, she lacked the skills required to be her former self. Perhaps being rude was the only choice she had for controlling her environment. Her rudeness certainly made waitresses go away.

Of course, not all suspect behavior of elderly people can be attributed to Alzheimer's disease. Most people have an embarrassing great aunt or uncle or grandma, who speaks too loudly because she cannot hear, who is tactless in her public commentary, or is simply old enough to no longer care about what other people think. For a short while, Mom's favorite expression was "I really don't give a damn." Her words were shocking because our real mom never swore. When Rhett Butler delivered the similar line, he was going for shock value. Sadly, Mother was offering extremely accurate self-analysis. We later learned that the last words dementia patients lose are swear words, sex talk, and racial slurs. The brain works hard to keep these words in a special file where they are guarded. With the onset of dementia, the guard is down and they are no longer off limits. So when that happens, these words are strangely accessible.

The change in her hygiene habits and personal grooming was alarming. Despite her former attention to good grooming, this new mother really didn't seem to care how she looked. As a teenager I had heard on numerous occasions, "Are you leaving the house in *that*?" This was not a request for information. It meant, "You march right back, young lady, and put on something presentable!" That she now didn't care about how she looked took great effort to understand. Had she forgotten how to be her true self?

When the family stopped to consider what was going on in her brain, we realized that she was not simply forgetting to bathe, to be kind, to be interesting and interested. She had lost the ability to organize and retrieve information that would enable her to act on her personal standards and expectations. We were jolted by the sharp contrast between her former self and this foul-smelling woman with a dirty bathrobe gathered around her body with a leather belt, her hair flying and tangled.

Each time one of us returned for a visit, the first thing we looked for was whether or not she had bathed. Most of the time she had not. Dad was quick to point out when she hadn't changed her clothes in many days. We worried about how he was dealing with this doppelgänger. We wanted her to bathe for his sake as much as for hers. He needed the woman who, even when she was going out to work in the flower beds early in the morning, started her day crisp and clean, wearing a shirt that matched the pants with just the right shoes, usually Keds. He needed his wife back just as much as we needed our mother back.

Although changes in Mother's appearance were disheartening, nothing was more startling than her frequent references to alcohol. She was quite obsessed. For all her life, Mother had scorned alcohol in any form. So I was surprised at her response one day when we were leaving for the shopping center and someone asked where we were going. Her reply was so out of character: "Going to get more vodka. We're out of it in my room." A car ride on a hot day would provoke, "Sure could go for a cold beer right now." She even attributed her frequent falls to being drunk. How odd to hear these words coming from the same mouth that would pucker in disdain at the mention of drinking.

We had no choice but to adjust to Mom's altered personality. After all, her lack of concern for her personal appearance and her jokes about drinking were really our problem not hers. Still, at times we wanted to say to her, "Who are you, and what have you done with our mother?"

CHAPTER 9

WASHING AWAY THE TANGLES

There must be quite a few things that a hot bath
won't cure, but I don't know many of them.
~ SYLVIA PLATH

I remember the smell of the Tame Cream Rinse my mother used to smooth away the tangles in my hair when I was a child in the 1950s. If only I had a potent bottle of Tame to wash away the tangles in my mother's brain, I could wash away this other woman and get my mother back.

This new woman was always in need of a bath. The fact that Mom would not bathe was a constant reminder of the problem. Each visit from my sisters or me included an attempt to get her into the shower.

Bathing was becoming frightening and confusing for her. She was resistant to and offended by the suggestion that she should bathe. She did whatever she could to get out of taking a shower. A bath in the tub had been ruled out because of the fear of her falling. She was resistant, even indignant, at the offer of help. She could do it herself. Unfortunately, she didn't do it herself, not even when we laid out the towel and wash cloth, her clean clothes, and started the shower running.

Once I watched my sisters at the closed bathroom door, so pleased that they had gotten Mom into the shower. I hated to burst their bubble, but my experiences had taught me that hearing the shower run did not mean Mom was showering. After a few minutes she turned off the water and called out, "I'm done." As steam rolled out, mother emerged from the bathroom. Her hair was still dry and matted; her washcloth and towel, still dry and folded on the vanity. She obviously was not clean, yet she insisted she had taken a shower. It didn't matter whether her insistence resulted from purposeful deception or loss of memory of how to take a shower. The situation was more complex than simply refusing to bathe.

We hypothesized about the reasons for her fears. Perhaps her long-term memory recalled soaking in a tub, not standing in a shower with streaming water attacking her. Early in her life she had not lived in houses with running water—an old-time phrase meaning a house did not have water plumbed into it. Mother's great-grandchildren would not recognize this old expression. I always lived in a house with plumbing, but I remember my great-grandparents' house with an outdoor toilet and a spring house from which we carried fresh water. The house I lived in as a child had a bathtub but not a shower, so I assume my mother did not live in a house with a shower until she was well into adulthood, and then it would have been a shower flowing into a bathtub and not a separate shower stall. Perhaps that was the problem. The once relaxing and soothing experience of a bath in a tub was too dangerous for her unsteady and less agile older body. There were no memories of taking a shower had she been able to recall the experience.

Adding safety bars to the shower stall eased some of our worries but probably did not address the worries she had. Other factors were at play. We learned that fear of bathing is common among Alzheimer's patients and is caused by a number of things. People with AD lose the ability to judge the depth of the water, so stepping into a tub produces anxiety. They also have difficulty distinguishing between a dark bath mat and a hole in the floor, so stepping out of a tub or a shower is frightening as well. Also there is the anxiety over loss of privacy and loss of control. Patients feel inadequate when they need help with a process that has been easy in the past. Some patients fear the water itself . . . or getting water or soap in their eyes . . . or the temperature of the water . . . the force of water coming from the faucet . . . the noises of splashing water and flushing toilets . . . the temperature of the room . . . being left alone in a room . . . being left alone in a room that no longer makes sense . . . .

In dealing with Mother's refusal to bathe, all of these possibilities needed to be considered in addition to the one clear cause. Her progressive brain deterioration meant she could no longer organize for the steps in the process that bathing required. There were so many things we didn't know how to handle. There were so many things we didn't know.

CHAPTER 10

TIME TO TALK ABOUT THE RESEARCH

Knowledge is power. Information is liberating.
Education is the premise of progress,
in every society, in every family.
~ KOFI ANNAN

We don't have to look too far back in history to find the time when people didn't live so long. The rise in diagnoses of Alzheimer's disease (AD) may be the result of people living long enough for the evidence of it to show up, just as the longer Grandpa lives, the more likely he is headed for a hip replacement. Not long ago, all cases of memory loss were lumped together under the category "senile dementia." The cause was attributed to what was called "hardening of the arteries."

Today, doctors use the term "dementia" to describe damage to brain cells. Dementia is not a disease itself, but a group of symptoms. These symptoms—including disruption of memory, thinking, and reasoning—occur when specific diseases or conditions are present. Dementia can be caused by AD, but it also can be caused by other things that damage brain cells—Parkinson's disease, Huntington's disease, vitamin B12 deficiency, stroke, drug abuse, or tumors (National Institute of Neurological Disorders, 2015).

So dementia is the large category of symptoms resulting from damage to the brain. Alzheimer's is a specific disease. AD is one type of dementia. It is a neurological disorder—a brain disorder—that interrupts the brain's ability to function normally. The cause of this interruption for a person with AD is very specific to this disease. Two things are happening in the brain of an AD patient: plaques and tangles. There is a buildup of sticky, insoluble proteins in the spaces between the nerve cells of the brain. These are beta-amyloid plaques. Second, there are tangled bundles of protein threads inside the nerve cells. These are neurofibrillary tangles made up of Tau protein. These plaques and tangles are markers of the disease, something like the way a runny nose is a marker of the common cold. Researchers have not identified the cause or causes of AD. They do know plaques on the outside of brain cells and tangles on the inside eventually result in irreversible damage (National Institute on Aging, 2015).

Some types of dementia can be reversed. For example, a brain tumor can be removed, blood flow to the brain can be restored, or a chemical imbalance can be stabilized. The kind of dementia caused by AD is progressive. AD is a terminal disease. It will not get better over time. Brain cells cease to communicate; tissue shrinks; damage spreads; cells die. The patient slowly loses the ability to retrieve memories and process information, eventually forgetting how to swallow, even how to breathe. The beginning point of plaques and tangles growing in the patient's brain is believed to precede its symptoms by many years (Norton, 2015).

Although AD is not reversible—at least not with current medication or technology—it is, however, treatable. The terms "treatable" and "curable" do not mean the same thing. For example, skin cancer and one type of glaucoma are highly curable. Diabetes and asthma are treatable diseases. Pneumonia can be cured, even though the common cold cannot be cured; but the common cold is treatable. Many diseases that cannot be cured can be controlled in ways that do not significantly disrupt the patient's daily life. People with diabetes take insulin; people with asthma use inhalers. In the case of polio, we can say that the polio vaccine has eliminated the disease in most of the world, so people consider polio to be cured when it has, in fact, been prevented. Some diseases are curable if caught in the early stages. Alzheimer's is not one of them. At least not yet.

Five drugs are currently approved by the US Food and Drug Administration for treating AD. Their brand names are Aricept, Razadyne, Exelon, Namenda, and Namzaric. These do not cure the disease or stop its progression. They treat its symptoms in that they may ease symptoms such as memory loss and confusion. The extent to which these drugs accomplish the task is difficult to judge. The amount of damage in the brain and the rate of progression of the disease varies from patient to patient. Another variable that makes efficacy unpredictable is that drugs are introduced to patients at differing stages of the disease along what already may be a highly individualized rate of progression. The functioning of the brain is complex, and scientists are just beginning to discover the mechanics of its electrical signals and chemical processes that create thoughts and store memories. Memory is not an organ that can be examined to determine its health.

The treatment of memory impairment is difficult to measure, unlike measuring high blood pressure, for example. There are tools for easily measuring blood pressure and assessing the drugs used to treat it when it's too high or low, but measuring memory is far more subjective and far more complex.

The hope in using these approved drugs is that introduction of them early—in the initial stages of memory impairment—will forestall the progression of the disease. There have been cases of modest improvement or slowed rate of decline, especially in the first months of delivery of the drugs (Alzheimer's Association, 2016b). There is no proof that they change the outcome of the disease.

One problem with treatment of AD using currently available drugs seems to be that there is no way to tell if progression of the disease would be greater if the patient had *not* been taking the drug. There is no control group for Grandma. Saying that Mom "seems less confused today" is hardly scientific analysis. Scientists are at the beginning level of understanding the complexities of the disease and the efficacy of the drugs used to treat it. At the present state of research, the most consistently observed—the most reliable—risk factor for getting Alzheimer's disease is living to be old.

Many anticipate breakthroughs in the understanding of the underlying factors that cause AD and sustain its progression. The present state of AD research is yielding slow but steady progress as one small discovery builds on the last small discovery—the pattern of most scientific research. Very few conclusions have been reached regarding what does not cause Alzheimer's disease. According to the Alzheimer's Association, researchers have concluded that AD is not linked to aluminum cookware or cans, flu shots, silver dental fillings, or the artificial sweeteners (Alzheimer's Association, 2016a).

An *AARP Bulletin* article laments the lack of funding for Alzheimer's research despite the rapid rise in the incidence of the disease (Reid, 2015). That article identifies two specific areas of research that could show promise. One area being explored notes that Down syndrome patients are likely to have plaques and tangles—the two signs considered evidence of Alzheimer's disease—early in life, in their teens or twenties. Yet they typically exhibit no dementia until middle age, or never, since the life expectancy is short for some Down syndrome patients. A better understanding of Alzheimer's disease may result from study of the plaques and tangles of these Down syndrome patients who do not have Alzheimer's disease, even though they have plaques and tangles.

The other study identified in the *AARP* article regards the discovery that patients who suffer with rheumatoid arthritis seldom develop dementia. Inquiry as to why this happens has focused on the kinds of medication taken by patients with rheumatoid arthritis, but even after extensive investigation of the medications for the disease, no conclusive link can be found between the medication and dementia.

Attempts to find cures for Alzheimer's disease have focused on ways to clear away beta-amyloid plaque. Studies of aducanumab, a monoclonal antibody that targets clumps of beta-amyloid in the brain, is the subject of recent investigation. Development of this antibody as a drug for the treatment of dementia, or any of the others being studied, will take years (Scuitti, 2016).

Some researchers studying Alzheimer's disease have shifted focus from the beta-amyloid plaques to the Tau tangles, investigating whether Tau protein is the main culprit that drives the process of declining cognitive function instead of beta-amyloid protein (Punsky, 2015). Studies are focusing on how, or if, Tau protein functions to protect the structure of brain cells, and whether the collapse of healthy brain cell structure—when those tangles show up —is the cause or the effect of changes in Tau protein (Lieff, 2015).

The painstaking research continues. As yet, the best results have led to drugs that treat the disease. A cure has proved elusive. A report from Mayo Clinic (Mayo Clinic Staff, 2016) confirms this assessment and offers some hope, saying that attempts to understand how the disease disrupts the brain may lead to treatments that alter the processes causing the disruption. The report discusses several paths of exploration: work on drugs that assist the immune system in preventing beta-amyloid plaques from clumping; studying a cancer drug that appears to turn off a protein in the body found to interact with beta-amyloid to destroy nerve cell connections; studying how to prevent Tau protein from tangling and collapsing the brain's communication system between cells.

Researchers from Massachusetts Institute of Technology (as cited in PubMed Health, 2016) have attempted to restore memories of mice bred to have a disease similar to Alzheimer's. By using light to stimulate synapses between nerve cells, they discovered that mice could respond using learned behavior recorded in memory that had been inaccessible previously because of the Alzheimer's-like condition. Mice in the control group did not show retrieval of memory.

Researchers at University of Minnesota (as cited in Lerner, 2016), have focused on a natural enzyme, caspase-2, which is believed to play a key role in dementia. Also using laboratory mice genetically altered to mimic Alzheimer's disease, researchers have discovered that lowering the enzyme results in reversing memory loss. They also say that human application of this discovery is a long way off, possibly as long as 10 years.

These studies are only a few of the complex areas of inquiry scientists continue to explore. They are given here as examples of the kinds of research in which scientists are engaged. The list of what we know for sure is short and incomplete; much awaits discovery. Many believe the breadth and depth of the research lags far behind the urgent need for more and better information regarding Alzheimer's disease and other types of dementia (Reid, 2015). The Alzheimer's Association projects that by 2050, the incidence of Alzheimer's disease in people over 65 will nearly triple (2016c).

In the meantime, treatments for Alzheimer's disease—other than drug therapies—include behavior modification by caregivers or any adaptive procedures that make the disease less onerous to the patient.

In early stages of dementia, it is hard to tell the difference between dementia caused by AD and dementia caused for other reasons. Nevertheless, AD is the most common form of dementia, estimated to make up 60% to 80% of the cases. The second highest incidence of dementia is vascular dementia, which often results after a stroke or series of strokes but can also result from any interrupted blood flow to the brain (World Health Organization, 2015).

People who are worried about declining memory skills should not assume they have Alzheimer's disease or any other kind of dementia. Just as not all tumors are cancerous, not all forgetfulness that accompanies old age is AD . . . or vascular dementia or frontotemporal dementia or Lewy body dementia or any of the other forms of dementia resulting from damage to the brain and significantly hindering daily life.

Some forgetfulness is a normal part of aging. Memory loss is not. Dementia caused by memory loss is more than forgetfulness because it makes independent life impossible. It takes away the ability to use language, reasoning, and logic. Forgetfulness may mean a person cannot recall the name of his nephew's newborn child or say the word that seems to be on the tip of her tongue. A person is forgetful if she stands with the refrigerator door open as if its contents need to be guarded while wondering what she's looking for. However, none of these lapses rob the person of the ability to later recall the name of the child, find the word she wants, or go back to the fridge to get the orange juice. With age, the body is not as agile as it once was, and the neural connections in the brain are not as fast. Some changes in memory and thinking skills occur even in healthy aging. Dementia is not a part of healthy aging.

Being forgetful may mean a person has a condition called mild cognitive impairment. This is a condition in which memory and thinking skills have declined beyond what is normal for the person's age or education. Many people with mild cognitive impairment may later be diagnosed with AD, but some will not. For that reason, it's important for a person to identify what is forgetfulness, what is mild cognitive impairment, and what is a more serious memory problem.

According to the Alzheimer's Association, one in three seniors in the United States die with AD or another kind of dementia (2016c). That does not mean these people die *from* AD or dementia. What it probably means is that a lot of people's grandmas were taken to the hospital from the nursing home because Grandma developed pneumonia, and she died there. Pneumonia was the last health event of her life. There's about a 30% chance that she died *with* dementia, most likely Alzheimer's disease. Which tool the grim reaper uses is of great consequence for those who do the important work of research, but it is of little consequence for families who deal with the passing of Grandma. To identify the reasons for death, families resort to what they can tell a five-year-old child: "Grandma died because she was very old. You are very young and Mommy and Daddy are young, and we will not die for a long time." And then they pray, "Let it be so."

CHAPTER 11

"TOO BAD YOU HAD TO PUT YOUR MOTHER IN A NURSING HOME"

> True freedom lies in the realization
> and calm acceptance
> of the fact that there may very
> well be no perfect answer.
> ~ ALLEN REID MCGINNIS

Sometimes concerned and kind people share information and opinions that are just not useful. I cringed every time someone said, "Your mom seems just fine to me." She was able to carry on a conversation; she was very present in the moment. Her inability to add new information to a conversation or think independently about a topic was barely noticeable by most people. She was never one to make verbal challenges or engage in philosophical discussions.

I understand the observation that most people made, however. People with Alzheimer's become very good at surface conversations, ones that do not venture far past the discussion of the weather or the repetition of what other people have just said. They can hide their inadequacies and fool lots of people.

In fact, some years ago I can remember wondering why one sweet old lady was in an Alzheimer's unit as I visited my step-grandmother, also a patient there. I was especially close to Grandma Norma. I lived 140 miles away and visited as much as

I was able. One time we were visiting at the kitchen table of the Alzheimer's care facility. We were engaged in a pleasant conversation. I tried to carry the burden of speech as much as I could and thus protect my grandmother from too many questions.

The subject was something that had happened in the distant past. The sweet elderly lady who sat with us often joined in, making reference to places mentioned or people I assumed both she and my grandmother knew. We were talking about my sister, Lori, who was someone special to Grandma Norma and her actual blood-related granddaughter. Lori, a beautiful and willful child, was born when I was sixteen. We were reminiscing, telling the well-worn family stories about how stubborn Lori was as a child. The woman, who had never met Lori, once again joined in our conversation, adding, "Oh, my, my, she was always like that." Minutes before I would have told the woman's family, "Your mom seems just fine to me." But that woman was not fine. Neither was Grandma Norma, and neither was Mother.

People who wondered about whether our mother should be in a nursing home had not seen her in a dirty bathrobe with unwashed hair and smelling like vomit. They did not know she confined herself to her room, seldom leaving it. They did not know she had long ago banished her husband to another part of the house. They did not know she would not take her medicine. They did not know about the time she could have burned down the house. They did not know her confusion and pain.

Her children came home to figure out what was to be done about our mother's sad situation. It was the first time the family faced the problem head on. We knew what we wanted. We wanted her to be safe, to bathe regularly, to take her medicine.

The thing about a difficult decision is that no easy and obvious answer presents itself. If the answers were obvious and the future easy to see, our family could have handled the problem. But families are fascinating—any difficult decision is layered with complexities. We believed our complexities were unique to our family, though that probably was not a reasonable assumption. I suspect that dysfunction in all families is part of the mix—only the specifics of the dysfunction are unique, not the fact of it.

Mother married my stepfather when I was twelve years old. He was not first choice of the three girls from her first marriage. The youngest of us was only nine years old and would have voted however we older two directed her. But our votes didn't count. We received the speech from Granny, Mom's mom, asking, "Don't you want your mom to be happy?" Of course we did; in fact, we had built our little lives upon the principle of being very good little girls. Yet only the youngest called Norm "Dad" because she remembered little about our real father—which was a blessing in many ways. The story of our father and the divorce is something I made peace with long ago. Parents don't always love us as much as we need but as much as they are able. But that's a different story.

Over the years, Pam and I came to understand the dedication and love it must have taken for Norm . . . Dad . . . to take on a pre-made family with a woman ten years older than he. Mother always looked much younger than her age. When they were first married, it didn't matter that much, but as she grew to be an older woman and Norm still seemed a relatively young man, I wondered how much the noticeable difference in their ages factored in the tension between them.

Then, with the onset of Alzheimer's, how much did the age difference play in her confusion about which man had harmed and betrayed her? Increasingly, Mom confused my real father with my stepdad. We first noticed this when she talked about Norm's '47 Ford pickup. That vehicle had belonged to my real father, not Norm. With the advantage of hindsight, we realized she was increasingly blaming Norm for our birth father's faults and inadequacies. Identifying her misplaced blame explained her attitude, but it did nothing to address the problems that ensued. The major one was that Norm—the stepdad of the older children and the father of the younger two—was unable to get our mother to bathe or to take her medicine.

Mother had told us girls that "when the time came," she didn't want to live with any of us. She used words like "not being a burden." And she might have meant she didn't want to be burdened by our fast-paced households. We knew she really meant that a nursing home was her choice. She made us promise. She was very specific about not wanting Norm to take care of her. In fact, she decided she wanted to be at the nursing home where our youngest sister worked. The staff at Lori's division of the facility knew Mom first not as a patient, but as Lori's mother, who brought them goodies at Christmas time. So Mom had a big part in our decision to seek care for her in a nursing home. The real struggle would be over *when* that would happen. Mother assumed the move to nursing care would be a long way off; we looked at her life and assumed some urgency.

The speed of her decline and all the things severely impacting her life pointed to nursing care as a solution. The fact that she had long-term care insurance made it financially possible. Then, after Mom spent a two-day stay in the hospital, a doctor advised that she be closely supervised.

No one recalls who first brought up the idea of looking for nursing care. I suppose that's a good thing. Much is unspoken in all families; contemplating the road not taken serves no useful purpose—at least not for our family. One would think that the time she could have burned down the house by forgetting the bacon cooking on the stove would have been the thing that started the nursing home discussion. But in the end, when people asked why we put our mother in a nursing home, every one of us went straight to one answer: She needed a bath.

We wanted Mom to have a good quality of life in the time she had left. We wanted her to live with a degree of dignity she certainly was not achieving at home. We wanted to give her a chance to be happy. For us, that started with social interaction, medicine on time, good food, and a bath. The choice became either finding a good nursing home for mom or allowing her to remain at home in the sad situation that wasn't working.

The first home we considered was the one Mom had picked out. When we walked down the residence halls of the facility, we saw slumping and slouching old people, many with blank stares. We didn't consider that these old people were getting social interaction, medicine on time, food, and baths. The stark reality is that nursing homes house old people. They take patients as they are and not as their families wish them to be. Ignoring that truth, we went in search of the shiny object—a nursing facility that matched our preferences . . . one with more cheerful-looking residents.

The place we found was lovely. Mother agreed because she toured it with us. We all decided this place could provide a setting in which we imagined her living with . . . we didn't know quite what . . . maybe it was living with greater ease. There was an atrium and library. It seems rather silly now to have imagined Mother reading all the classics she never got around to while raising five children. No one actually said that would happen, but the possibility was hanging there silently in the mix of emotions, rational and irrational thoughts, assumptions and suppositions clouding the process of decision making.

This was a newly built facility—a significant point because, without the presence of needy old people, we were allowed to imagine the place populated with elderly people who were clean and content . . . happy people, who were as pleased as punch to have advanced to their golden years. We were not accounting for the nature and the conditions of aging. It would have been helpful if the doctor had let the family know what we were in for . . . the long struggle ahead for Mom . . . Mom, with her strong bones and strong heart.

The nursing facility we selected was a beautiful setting with all the amenities we imagined she would enjoy. We did not understand the nature of the disease with which we were dealing. What we wanted for her was an impossibility. Finding a great setting to accommodate the future we imagined for her would not make that future happen. Location does not postpone mental decline caused by Alzheimer's disease. Neither does it avert the consequences.

Mother stayed at this facility for over a year. Looking back, we can only hope the beautiful setting gave her joy. I know that for quite some time she liked the restaurant-style dining room where she sat with interesting people who seemed not to know that she repeated her stories.

After a year we moved Mother to the facility where our sister worked—the location Mom had suggested in the first place. There were several reasons for the move—not the least of which was her continuing decline. Another important reason was that Lori was carrying most of the responsibility as the family's advocate for Mom, and the move made it easier for her since she was in the building. The move changed Mother's circumstances very little.

I guess our family tacitly decided not to look back. As I write this, it occurs to me that it's the first time any of us have thought about how we made the decision. Perhaps lots of people look back on life, seeing where their range of choices narrowed to just a few—none of which provided them with exactly what they wanted. It's a sorrowful thing to have regrets. It's also a waste of time and emotional energy. We based our decisions on the options we saw in front of us.

CHAPTER 12

FIRST NIGHT IN THE NURSING HOME

Some days there won't be a song
in your heart. Sing anyway.
~ EMORY AUSTIN

The move into the first nursing facility to serve as Mother's home became a reality at the beginning of a new year. It was cold. The emotional climate at the house she was leaving and where Dad would continue to live was dark, damp, and heavy.

We moved her in with speed and efficiency. I don't remember stopping to evaluate how Mom reacted. I'm pretty sure she didn't realize she would be staying. All her daughters were there, so I assumed she was content . . . and trusting. The day blurs in my memory. One of the few things I specifically recall is that a nurse put the wrist bracelet on her—the one that sets off an alarm in case she tried to leave the building. Mom looked at the bracelet with her name on it. "But I can just tell them my name," she said. I don't recall responding to her. In the emotion of that moment I couldn't think about it too deeply.

Now I rationalize the concession. Mother's new bracelet meant she was in a world of uniformity—a world with rules imposed upon her because at some point in the future, patients in her condition could be expected not only to wander off but also to forget their names. Mother had never been a wanderer, but the rules were applied to her and all residents regardless of individual personalities. My mother had to wear a wrist bracelet, even though she probably would not wander off, because someone else's mother might. What Mother received for that imposition was the absence of steps to fall down, meals cooked and served to her, and a bath twice a week.

We had already begun the task of sorting through Mother's life to find which things to take from her spacious home to her new and narrowed life. Envelopes, nail clippers, cosmetics—all things she too soon would not need . . . or, more accurately stated, things she too soon would not be able to use—were packed up and moved along with her. So many of the items were like the little sewing kit I've always taken on vacation and never used—its only purpose to give me a sense of being prepared.

Dad was part of the move; he knew he needed to help. If we were anxious about the task before us, how was our dad handling it? While we were busy moving her into the nursing home, he was overwhelmed with the reality of moving her out of their home. Moving his wife meant she would no longer be in the chair across the room from him—ever. It had to be heart wrenching. We could tell he would rather be anywhere else, even though we had talked about this step in Mom's care and well being and all had agreed this move was the best choice.

To avoid standing around looking uncomfortable, Dad busied himself moving Mother's favorite recliner next to her bed and hooking up her television and telephone. He fussed over getting the new flat screen TV at just the right angle and hiding the numerous TV and phone cords because that was easy to do. He was the guy working on repairs, not the husband moving his wife into a nursing home. On this day, the only way he could cope was to disengage himself from the decision. Someone else had started this, someone else must be guilty, and some other person was starting the heartache that was sure to follow. When there were no more tasks for him to do, he stood in the doorway confused and conflicted, the tears starting to flow.

Debbie knew it was time to take him home. She later told us he cried all the way back to the house. It was done. As he sat in his chair looking at the empty space where Mom's recliner had been, he said, "I don't know how I let you kids talk me into this." He said this without animosity. After he physically separated himself that day from his wife of almost 50 years, he occasionally—then seldom—visited her. The burden of his sadness was so great that he never went back to her emotionally.

I don't know how we came to the decision for Pam and me to stay with Mom that first night at the nursing home. We did not ask permission from the staff. We operated on the principle that it's easier to beg forgiveness than to ask permission.

Pam curled up with Mom on the bed as I settled into the large reclining chair. I remember Mom laughing a bit at our presence. We didn't know what she was thinking about the whole thing but assumed she was comforted by our presence. During the night she woke several times to ask, "Where are we?" It was the question we were there to answer.

It's strange now to recall that we never answered her specific question. We answered a different question. "We are here, Mom. It's OK." Each time it was answer enough. She was glad we were there, and the next morning she told us that. We didn't know whether or not she understood the reality of the move from her home. We talked about it in vague generalities. I'm guessing at that point her mind was still operating well enough to know what was going on.

Mom's first night passed without collapse of the universe, and the next day the nurse came to us and said, "You girls are going to have to go home and let us do this." The nurse gave us permission to let go. Mother would stay in nursing care facilities—first this one and later the one she had originally picked out— until her request to go home no longer meant she wanted to go back to her house.

CHAPTER 13

B-I-N-G-O

> Humor is just another defense
> against the universe.
> ~ MEL BROOKS

One brick shy of a full load, one fry short of a happy meal, one synapse short of a memory—any funny metaphor used to denote lack of mental prowess falls flat when faced with the reality of a humorless situation.

We watched our mother's slow decline, puzzled by the random nature of the disease's advance. At times, she seemed perfectly lucid. She remembered details of the distant past with clarity; a few minutes later, she repeated the same details as new information.

Our preconceived notion was that memory loss would be steady and gradual. And perhaps if we chart the decline in a rear view mirror that might be the observable reality, but in real time, it was not the case. Clarity surfaced and vanished randomly. What amazed us most was that Mom never lost her cleverness. After her move to the care facility, she was quite popular with the staff, and we assumed it was because of her quick—though repetitious—wit. The nurses seemed delighted by her antics, a regular stand-up comedy routine "appearing nightly" . . . weekly . . . monthly. They joked with her, using standard responses to her inevitable commentary. Perhaps they liked her because they were trained to be attentive and were good people.

We wondered what was going on in her head. What prompted her to joke consistently with the meds nurse about being the local pill-pusher yet fail to access information about what day it was or whether she had eaten lunch? How was she dealing with why she was in a nursing home? She must have formed an opinion, possibly assuming we thought she was a little crazy because one time, she pointed out the resident who was walking past us using walking aids like ski poles to steady herself. "You think *I'm* crazy," she said. "She thinks she's skiing." Sometimes we knew exactly what she was thinking, as when she looked in the mirror, startled, and said, "What the heck happened here?" Even as the disease progressed, she could animate a group of people by delivering a good line. At her granddaughter's wedding reception, she had everyone at her table laughing when the salad course was served. It was beautiful—exquisitely arranged on the plate. Her observation: "I don't know whether to eat it or wear it."

Much like the children of all families with failing parents, we met our problems with the skills we had. Our familial instinct was to resort to humor as a coping mechanism. The first time all of us visited Mother after she moved to the nursing home was for Tuesday night bingo. Nursing home bingo is pain-ful-ly slow. For us, a dose of humor defended against the emotional chaos we were feeling. Watching elderly people play bingo in a nursing home was too depressing to be taken seriously, but it was good to be together laughing again with Mom. I'm not sure our middle sister, Pam, was there, but I want her to have been there, so she agrees to remember the events of the bingo session as they are told here.

BINGO IN THE NURSING HOME: A SHORT COMEDY IN A PARTIAL SCENE

Cast of Characters: Family members—MOM and her CHILDREN (REGINA, PAM, DEB, BARRY, LORI). Nursing Home ACTIVITY DIRECTOR. BINGO CALLER. Bingo Players: EDNA, MARTHA, RALPH, THELMA, FRED, and additional BINGO PLAYERS in various stages of alertness.

[A well-lit activity room of a comfortable and spacious nursing home. On either side of the doorway to the hall, bulletin boards announce activities of the month, display notices, and offer posters of encouragement and motivation. Opposite the door are three large floor-to-ceiling windows and an emergency exit door. Seven tables are set up for bingo. Gray-haired residents are assembled in the room as others shuffle in. Some are ambulatory, but others use walkers or wheelchairs. Enter MOM and her CHILDREN, who seat themselves at the back table.]

CALLER. OK. Let's get this show on the road. We're playing for quarters this week. Is everybody ready? [*Murmurs from the crowd. Few people are ready.* ACTIVITY DIRECTOR *assists in distribution of bingo cards: one card to most players, several cards to some. Bingo players stop to stare suspiciously at* MOM *and* CHILDREN, *who quickly learn they should take only one card each.* MARTHA *takes all remaining cards from the box.* CALLER *begins the game.*]

CALLER. Under the B. 14.

EDNA. Wait, wait!

RALPH. Didn't anyone make the popcorn? [*Bingo game stops while all watch unidentified young person make the popcorn.*]

CALLER. Under the G. 47.

EDNA. [*Loudly*] Did he say 47?

MARTHA. [*Disgusted*] No, he said G 47.

ACTIVITY DIRECTOR. [*Loudly*] Edna, do you have your hearing aid in today?
RALPH. Did he call 7?
MARTHA. No, Edna, don't put the chip on 37. [*Shouting*] 47!
EDNA. Oh . . . h . . . ! Wait, wait!
FRED. There's no damn 37 under the G! [ACTIVITY DIRECTOR *approaches* FRED. *Whispers in his ear regarding language use violation.*]
CALLER. Under the O. 73.
[*Thelma begins to sing* "Blessed Assurance."]
EDNA. Hold your horses. You're going too fast.
CHILDREN. [*Various murmuring sigh*] Ahhh . . . Ugh . . .
EDNA. Wait, wait!
BARRY. [*Aside to other children, whispering*] Jesus, Edna, get with the program!
CALLER. Under the O. 68.
[*Bingo interrupted while popcorn is served.*]
CALLER. Under the B. 11. [*Bingo players concentrate on their cards.*]
REGINA. [*Whispering to siblings.*] See how this works? Pretty serious. Under no circumstances do we need to win.
BARRY. [*Whispering. Placing a handful of quarters on the* table.] We could make side bets. You know, have a bingo win just on our cards. And I'll bet a quarter Martha strangles Edna with her bib. [CHILDREN *muffle giggles.*]
PAM. [*Also whispering.*] I'll bet we don't get out of here until midnight! [CHILDREN *laugh.*]
DEB. [*Also whispering.*] I'll bet two quarters Jim over there falls asleep before the end of this game.
LORI. Oops. Too late. Sweet dreams, Jim. [*More laughing by MOM's children.*]
MOM. [*Suppressing her own laughter, but with scolding tone.*] You kids, shush!
PAM [*Sputtering laugh, standing*] Where's the bathroom? Fast.

LORI. Well, they do have plenty of Depends around this place.
[*MOM's* CHILDREN *try to suppress contagious laughter. Cover mouths to stifle gasps for breath.*]
BARRY. [*Unable to avoid deep-throated laughter.*] Can we all just sing "Blessed Be the Tie That Binds" and be done.

[*Bingo game continues . . . etc., etc. . . . .*]

Although Mother was suppressing laughter of her own, her attempts to quiet us failed, much as they had when she hushed us in church. When we were young, she would turn from the pew in front of us to whisper, "You kids, stop it." Back then, she meant it. At the bingo game that day, she wasn't serious. Later, after Mom no longer recognized her children, she might have been truly annoyed by our laughter that day. She might have called it disrespect for the nursing home residents instead of feigning the reprimand. But her smile and her laughter told us she was pleased with her fun-loving children. She was not yet identifying with residents of the home. Her allegiance was still with us. She was still the mom, and we were her precocious children huddled around the kitchen table playing a game together. Finding humor in the bingo session separated us from the heartache that was nursing home bingo and all of the losses it implied.

Over the years, we discovered our family laughed more in the nursing home than other visitors. But maybe they laughed privately and we laughed publicly. Or, maybe we didn't notice other people's laughter, not being privy to what they found humorous in their lives. Mostly, they seemed sadder than we did. I wondered if they knew that a laugh can be as cleansing as a cry.

With her humorous nature serving as a constant, Mother's hit-or-miss memory became bearable. So every time we heard her say something like, "If you put on a necklace, they won't ask why you're still in your pajamas," we knew our real mother was still in there. What we didn't know was whether catching these glimpses of our mother made us happy to see her once more or served to exacerbate the pain of losing her again.

CHAPTER 14

CAREGIVERS: THE PROBLEM OF HIGH EXPECTATIONS

> It is a common observation that those who
> dwell continually upon their expectations
> are apt to become oblivious to the
> requirements of their actual situation.
> ~ CHARLES SANDERS PEIRCE

As the days wore on, Mother's life in the nursing home became tolerable. The family accepted it as the way of things. Mother was no longer checking in to offer her opinion on the matter.

Perhaps our gradual acceptance came because Mom accepted it, perhaps because she no longer mentioned home, or perhaps because we could no longer sustain the guilt. Now our major concern no longer centered on how she was feeling about the loss of control over her life. New permutations of old issues were in front of us.

Failure to bathe was the issue that had landed her in the ultimate time out. Although shifting daily responsibility to trained professionals made life easier for the family, that shift didn't mean that life was fine for her or staff members simply because someone had now scheduled her for bath time on Wednesdays and Saturdays. She wasn't exactly saying, "You mean I skipped my bath last time. I'll just get right up and take charge of that!"

Only after Mother looked as bad off as other severely ill residents did the nursing staff realize she had not and would not take a bath or shower without help.

Although the staff was trained in Alzheimer's care, they were not working in a facility specifically for Alzheimer's patients. Mom was in a typical nursing care facility. She had the legal right to refuse baths, and the staff treated her as if she still had the ability to make wise decisions. During the first months, she simply outwitted staff members by saying, "Just put the towel right there. I'll get to it when *Wheel of Fortune* is over" or "I took a sponge bath this morning." They were busy, overworked people and probably wanted to believe this was true. She probably believed it was true as well. After all, she was not refusing to be clean. Her progressive brain deterioration meant she could no longer recall having taken a bath. We needed to remember that. The staff needed to learn it. Convinced that our expectation of basic hygiene could be accomplished, we became increasingly frustrated with the staff's failure to solve the bathing dilemma.

The frustration regarding bathing built up over time until, on one particular day, Debbie was at wit's end. Having planned to take Mom out for a special event, she arrived at the nursing home to discover that, although Mom was dressed, she had not bathed. She smelled bad, and her hair was as mess. On her night stand lay a fresh towel and washcloth. Upset by how many times Mother had been trusted to bathe without assistance, Debbie searched the room finding sets of towels and washcloths in her dresser, in the closet, and even in the bookcase—11 sets of them, all unused. She marched down to the nurses' station, plopped the towels down on the desk, and steadied her voice to ask, "When is the last time my mother had a bath?" The nurse turned to a large folder and told her that Mother's bath days were Wednesdays and Saturdays.

"Yes," she replied, "I know when her baths are scheduled. What I need to know is whether or not she actually had a bath or shower at the scheduled time." She wanted to scream, "Can't you just do this one thing!" But she refrained as the nurse promised to discover whether or not Mom had bathed. When she returned to the room to propose a bath, she found Mom in bed.

"I wish you people would just leave me alone," Mother responded as she turned to the wall. At that point Debbie had become one of "you people," instead of her daughter. She stepped outside the room, braced her back against the wall, and slowly slid down it, as she started to cry. She needed to leave. Not wanting any of the nurses to see her, she forced herself to stand and she headed for the door, increasing her stride as she traveled the hall. She was almost running when she passed a second nurses' station, waving off the nurse with whom she sometimes chatted.

Near the exit door, she met another nurse who often cared for Mom. The nurse looked away; neither of them wanted to make eye contact. The nurse was dressed in her coat and apparently waiting for someone to pick her up. Debbie was startled by how sad she looked. No longer on duty and no longer having to deal with Mother's problems, this compassionate caregiver obviously had problems of her own. At that moment my sister saw her as a person whose life existed separate from our mother. She wondered about the worries of this nurse's life. She wondered if she waited for a ride while her car was being fixed. She wondered if she worried about the repair bill. She wondered if she were going home to an aging mother of her own who could not afford to be in this nursing home.

How easy—how selfish—it was for our family to fall into the trap of assuming our mother was the only patient who commanded the attention of people who tirelessly cared for her. They had a hard job to do, the turnover in workforce was high, and I'm sure the compensation could not match their efforts. Almost none of them knew the woman our mother had been. A few staff members had known Mother when she first arrived there, but after a while the nursing home staff knew her as an old woman—sometimes congenial, sometimes cranky—like all the other old and slumping and needy women in various stages of decline.

It was clear our high expectations were not doing Mom any good. We needed to encourage the staff to attend to her hygiene—the need we had been unable to meet at home. The nursing home was staffed with people trained to do that, who wanted to give her good care. We needed to let them care for her the best they could. They could focus on her needs, unburdened by memories of the person Mom had been and without emotional reaction to her transformation. Debbie was relieved when her dear friend cut through the emotional clutter and succinctly summed up the situation when she said, "Their job is to give her a bath. Your job is to love her."

CHAPTER 15

OBSERVING THE STEADY DECLINE

> There are things I can't force. I
> must adjust. There are times
> when the greatest change needed
> is a change of my viewpoint.
> ~ DENIS DIDEROT

The bathing dilemma resolved itself but not without drama. The family eventually decided to readjust expectations. Mother should be clean enough to be healthy and avoid infections. She was happy enough in the moment that was her entire reality. Eventually we no longer cringed when we saw her sock-less, with shoes on the wrong feet, and chocolate milk spilled down the front of her blouse. It was no longer unusual to see her in late afternoon wearing a pajama top with a fancy shirt worn over it. We were able, after a while, to consider her dress an interesting wardrobe choice. She was still making her own choices, which favored dark colors to hide the stains. Mom didn't need to be so clean that she sparkled just for the sake of making us feel better.

We also tried to do our part. The nurses appeared genuinely grateful when we offered to give Mom a bath occasionally. Of course, they could have been humoring us. We selected times when the bathing room was not busy, and after receiving instructions on the walk-in style tub, we tried to avoid bothering the nurses. The room designed for geriatric patients was much better than the situation at home, making the task much easier. My sisters and I joked about Mother having a spa experience. Any of us would have loved to de-stress with a soak in a tub like that one. What we knew, but didn't mention, was that a personal spa just down the hallway in a nursing home was not a fair exchange for lack of privacy and loss of freedom.

When giving baths at the nursing home, we had the luxury of time—something the nursing staff did not have. Also, we knew her personality and she trusted us, so we were better able to divert her attention. Assisting with bathing duties was good time spent with Mother not only because she got a bath, but also because it gave us insights into the progression of the disease that was now controlling her, something we might not have learned from sitting with her in her room. Experiencing the bathing episodes gave us a yardstick for measuring the decline that was happening in all parts of her life.

Much too often we failed to identify the disease as the cause for her troubles with bathing. To us, she was obstinate; she was just being difficult. Later, as skills quickly declined, it became easier to blame her diseased brain and not *her*. We learned to separate Mother from the disease.

As Mother's understanding of her condition dwindled, ours grew. It not only grew, but it also shifted over time in that discovering a solution to any specific problem did not mean our solution was applicable to the next problem. This shifting understanding of the extent of her problem paralleled her progressive decline. The more she went downhill, the more we recognized why. For example, we knew right away that she could not follow our instructions while bathing. We came to realize that she was probably missing words or the ability to hold in her brain the meaning of some of our words. At first, it was some of the words, then more, and then most of them. She also gradually lost ability to interpret abstract meaning. Eventually she could no longer be cajoled by a clever metaphor or subtle intent.

Non-verbal communication stays intact for people with Alzheimer's for a very long time. We can confirm this is true because in the late stages she would not respond to "You need to lift your arm, Mom." Yet if we lifted an arm, she knew to lift hers. We learned to give her a washcloth to busy her hands so that she could be a participant instead of a victim of the bath. Then, there was the importance of figuring out what she really wanted, regardless of what she seemed to be saying.

We knew that asking Mom if she was ready for her bath alerted her to the plan and set up the battle of resistance. At this particular time, back when Mom still knew who we were, my sister was able to coax and plead until she got Mom into the bath. Mom was uncooperative, an unwilling participant in every part of the process, but still showed her characteristic humor. Debbie was pushing up the sleeves of her red Wisconsin sweatshirt as she prepared to wash Mom's hair. Mom, to show her displeasure at being managed, looked up at her out of the corner of her eye and said, "I never liked Wisconsin." Later, Mom—a Notre Dame fan—would not be able to connect the red sweatshirt to the University of Wisconsin basketball or remember her sports preferences. She would not remember her grandson Jim graduated from the University of Wisconsin or how they had sat together cheering on the Badgers. She became more compliant at bath time once the language of resistance was not available to her and no smart remarks served her purpose. Next, after it made no difference who gave her a bath, she became physically aggressive, scratching nurses until they bled. She was scared and confused, and there were no words to encompass the enormity of her fear.

Once when I was there to give Mom a bath—after she had completely lost her short-term memory but could still talk about things from long ago—we strolled down to the bathing room as if taking a casual walk. I seated her in the tub, closed the door and turned on the water. Temperature of the water was very important to her; she had a narrow range of acceptable temperatures. I talked to her about the time when she was giving the oldest three daughters a bath. I recalled standing on the commode being dried off when I was about five years old. I fell into the window frame, and I cut my arm on a Venetian blind. I showed her the scar, which was then barely recognizable. She traced the scar with her finger and I believed she was trying very hard to remember.

As the warm, steamy air and sweet scent of bath soap encased us like a cocoon, Mom became compliant and loving as we talked. She was afraid someone would walk in. I locked the door, although I knew that was probably not a good idea. She spoke in a whisper, saying, "Let's just stay in here." I wondered where she was in time . . . what memories were still in her head.

The nursing staff, too, learned more about Mom's condition as time went on. They knew they could not depend on her to bathe on her own. They assigned someone to assist whenever she was bathed. The staff continually struggled with her refusals. They could not forcibly dunk her into water.

In addition to the issue of coaxing her into a bath, there was also the problem of who from the staff was going to give her a bath. Personnel assignment was an important matter if a person looked at the situation totally through Mom's point of view. Mother and her generation assumed male doctors and female nurses. When the young Hispanic man arrived to give her a bath, Mom was scared. She had too many other shocking changes going on in her life to deal with issues of gender role inclusiveness and ethnic diversity. Societal changes that her grandchildren would not give a second thought must have seemed one more frightening change in a world she could no longer interpret and through which she could no longer maneuver. Asking her to be led down the hallway to her bath by this young man must have been just as alarming to her as having someone give her an iPad and asking her to order lunch.

The young man was compassionate and skilled, respectful of her modesty. The fact that he did, indeed, give her a bath without incident is demonstration not only of his skill and compassion but also his patience and respect. Other staff members also deserved praise for their efforts. They understood that even though she had lost the ability to command respect, she still had the desire to be respected.

Trying to see the world from Mom's point of view was a scary proposition, even when looking closely at the very narrow topic of bathing. Imagine the fright at taking a bath when you can't trust your balance and you've lost depth perception. Imagine your physical and mental limitations in buttoning your shirt if your brain is losing ability to interpret tactile messages . . . if your fingers no longer seem to be at the end of your arms . . . if the mysterious buttons have no discernible relationship to the buttonholes.

It makes me feel sad, and I have to stop thinking and do something else for a while.

CHAPTER 16

DINING IN SLOW MOTION

> Lord, bless this food to the
> nourishment of our bodies,
> and our bodies to thy service.
> ~ A MEALTIME PRAYER

Watching a dining room full of elderly patients eat their meals was particularly depressing. It was dining in slow motion. All the more reason, I suppose, for residents to arrive early at the dining hall to get a head start on the arduous process. Sadly, for most of the people at my mother's table, mealtimes were the highlight of the day. They were greeted and directed to their places by cheerful staff who appeared to be happy to see them—even the grumpy and demanding ones.

Once Mother was in nursing care, we were delighted that she would get regular meals providing a healthy variety of foods from which she could choose. Ironically, she always chose the same things. The situation was still an improvement over her forgetting to eat at all or eating the third piece of lemon meringue pie because she could not remember having eaten the first slice or the second one.

We also hoped she would get intellectual stimulation by gathering around a table and talking with people her own age. We didn't consider how odd it must have felt for her to sit among these women—mostly women—forced together without the bonds of friendship or history or children to raise or church dinners to plan. Despite our desire for her to be part of satisfying and witty discussions, the talk at the table was always limited to safe subjects and comments on the immediate and obvious. There was no discussion of where they were when the boys—brothers, husbands, friends—returned from World War II. There was seldom a reference to exciting places they had visited or predicaments of life they had encountered.

Perhaps their conversations were different . . . better . . . when my sisters and I were not there to remind them of their children and the world they had left on the outside. I hoped so. At that point our family was still operating with a certain amount of naiveté, or maybe it was still outright denial.

I wondered what I would be like in 20 years. Would I initiate a discussion of my first experience of using a computer? Would I talk about being a working mother? Would I bring up my reaction to the treatment of soldiers returning from Vietnam? Probably not. Maybe I, too, would be tired and move slowly.

At least Mother was engaging in conversation—banal conversation—but conversation nonetheless. Later, after shallow conversation could not sustain a dialogue that allowed the worlds of the table mates to intersect, the exchanges collapsed from talk with others at the table to suspicions of others at the table. Each aging person moved into her own private bubble. These women were no longer the main characters of their own life stories. Later still, only silence and slow lifting of the spoon to the mouth.

After Mother had been in the nursing care facility for a while, we dropped the expectation of intellectual stimulation and focused on her intake of nourishment. A healthy appetite was followed by no appetite at all and followed next by simple failure of the mechanics of eating. Eventually the brain's signal to muscles that make the jaws rotate and grind food failed to communicate. We first noticed this when Mother would remove food from her mouth and place it on the side of her plate. At first it was dense meats; later the husky, outer layer of peas was beyond her ability to chew.

I wanted to make sure she was eating enough to keep her going, which didn't take much considering her inactive, almost lethargic lifestyle. I resorted to scooping up a forkful of mashed potatoes and placing it at the lower edge of her plate. I was surprised that she would pick up the fork and put it in her mouth. A spoonful of pudding, a fork with green beans—whatever food I placed near the right-hand edge of her plate—was eaten. The waiting fork must have signaled to her brain the need to complete the next step. I was pleased to see her eat, but in the back of my mind I knew this was a frightening precursor of what would come later: the need for her to be spoon-fed, participating only by opening her mouth and trying to chew. And after that, the disease would rob her of the memory of how to swallow.

I thought about tricks I had used to get my children to eat vegetables. "How old are you?" I would ask my daughter.

"Four!" she would proudly announce, holding up four fingers.

"Then you must eat four pieces of broccoli before you are finished." She was eager then to gobble up four pieces.

I had shared that story with Mother and would have shared it again. We could have laughed about it, but she could no longer remember family stories and, at that point, may not have remembered my daughter. She couldn't connect immediate circumstances to stories of the past. There could be no joke about her eating 87 pieces of broccoli, and she could not take solace in the knowledge of things having come full circle. You feed your daughter and then your daughter feeds you. She had lost so many things. I left Mother that day wishing she could understand that someone still cared if she ate her vegetables.

CHAPTER 17

"ALL I HEARD WAS SAWDUST AND SLEEP"

Night has brought to those who sleep,
only dreams they cannot keep.
~ ENYA BRENNAN, "PAINT THE SKY WITH STARS"

As I sat by Mother's bed and watched her sleep, I wondered about the dream world reality in which her mumbled words might make sense. Her sleep was shallow. She drifted deeper into sleep but soon after struggled to open her eyes.

I coughed and then she was awake and smiled at me, only to float off again as she whispered, "So many kids." Her own five children? The ones she taught in Sunday school? The poor starving children of Africa who would perish if we did not finish our dinners?

She returned to unintelligible mumbling and then blurted out with some urgency, "No, come back." I suspected her dream was not one of happier times. It was not about sitting down to Sunday dinner of Granny's fried chicken or a trip to catch butterflies in the Redwood Forest. What goes on in people's brains during sleep? Scientists know that when we sleep we are not just wasting time; the brain is very active. One theory is that sleep facilitates the body's restorative functions, allowing it to recover from the work it has done during waking hours. The dreaming stage—the REM sleep stage—is considered important in memory and learning. If only dreams could restore all of her brain's functions.

What happens in the memory-impaired brain of a sleeping Alzheimer's patient? So many mysteries. If only her dreams could go back to a happy time of the distant past. She might relive her teenage years and mischievous adventures. Perhaps she might recall the time she and her best friend left her grandparents' house for the evening, promising to be back between 10:00 and 11:00. As they left, they christened the front-yard tree on the left as "10:00" and the one on the right as "11:00." I chuckled as I recalled her old stories.

She became restless, fumbling with the covers as if attempting to fasten a row of buttons. Her hands stopped moving and inexplicably she said, "All I heard was sawdust and sleep."

Finally, there was a heavy sigh and then peaceful, soft snoring. I let out a deep sigh, too, unaware that I had been holding my breath.

CHAPTER 18

MOTHER'S MOVE TO EASY-CARE KNITS

All the art of living lies in a fine mingling
of letting go and holding on.
~ HAVELOCK ELLIS

P am stared into Mother's small closet at the nursing home. "These don't look like Mother's clothes," she announced. Lori and I exchanged glances; we knew exactly what she meant. Stretchy waistbands, sweatshirt-type tops, no-iron clothing in polyester and easy-care knit material. Her closet was filled with clothing that could be easily laundered and easily donned.

There were no crisp, white cotton shirts with French cuffs, no stylish ones with intricate embroidery of hummingbirds on the pockets. Now her clothes had no backbone; they were limp and slouchy. She would not search through her jewelry box for her favorite clunky jewelry to complete her outfit because—well, nothing could fashion-rescue a dull pink sweat suit.

"Well, they're her clothes now." I was simply acknowledging the sad truth.

We were removing summer clothes, ones that no longer fit or ones that were stained and replacing them with clothing better suited for the coming cold weather. We didn't discuss how seldom she was out of the building to experience the shift in seasons. We talked about her wardrobe as if she were not in the room.

"What are you girls doing over there?" This was when she was still able to perceive that our lowered tone of voice meant something.

"Just straightening this closet. Making sure your clothes match."

"Oh, it doesn't much matter," she replied. The problem exactly!

I remember when we were teenagers, and we displeased her by dashing off to church on a Sunday morning without much attention to how we looked. We had listened dutifully to sermons over the years and accepted the message of unconditional love, unconditionally. For meeting our classmates at the big game or other school events on Saturday night, we felt we had to work harder on our appearance. We scheduled time for the single bathroom, primped mercilessly, and experimented with the tiny bit of make-up we were allowed. She couldn't help but notice the contrast of our half-hearted attempts to be presentable for Sunday morning services. But we were young and we really didn't have to try so hard in those days. Besides, Saturday night's routine was more about applying attitude than applying hairspray.

We didn't understand until years later—probably after we had children of our own—how much Mother was invested in her children as a reflection of her value and competence as a homemaker. It was a different time. Her smart, well-behaved, perfectly groomed children filing into the pew beside her were symbols—representations of her worth and accomplishment as a mother: the most important job in the world. Back then, we didn't understand her complaints about our unenthusiastic efforts to dress up for church.

Now, so many years later, we riffled through her clothing, trying to find something for her to wear for a day out so people would know we didn't let our mother look like someone we had picked up at a homeless shelter. I don't recall what we made her struggle to get into, but I'm pretty sure it was not the pink sweat suit.

CHAPTER 19

WHAT ROLE FOR THE HUSBAND AND SON?

> A man may work from sun to sun, but
> a woman's work is never done.
> —ANONYMOUS, POSSIBLY DATING
> FROM REVOLUTIONARY WAR TIMES

Most women take charge of the home front. Someone, after all, must write the thank-you notes, know when the family is running low on peanut butter, remember Aunt Wilma's birthday, and make sure the kids' gym clothes are washed for Tuesdays and Thursdays. That person is usually, though not always, the wife. My experience is that the mom doesn't have to do it all; her job is to see that it all gets done. The assumptions of Generation Xers and Millennials might be different.

I have friends who will compliment my husband on the perfect doneness of the steaks he has placed on and taken off the grill. None of them, however, are so slow as to be oblivious to the fact that I have selected and purchased the steaks, prepared and applied the marinade—remembering to turn them occasionally, planned and prepared all the other dishes to be served, gotten a head start on the cleanup, and handed a platter of steaks to my husband, who captains the grill as he awaits praise.

I don't mind doing the kitchen work; I'm good at it. And I don't plan to change the oil in my car anytime soon. My husband is better at that, though I could learn to do that job if I wanted to assume another one. Division of labor is a good plan for running a household.

The problem is with the unequal value assigned to "men's work" versus "women's work." But that's a different discussion for another time. I bring up the issue here because division of labor and gendered role assignments are pertinent to the work of caregiving for elderly parents. Caring for others is largely women's work. Women, by a wide majority, fill the ranks of elementary teachers and nurses. It's not that men cannot do these jobs well; it's just that men of past generations were not trained for or expected to learn the skills of caregiving.

That could be changing. I know of many young husbands who change their children's diapers. That's something their fathers did occasionally and their grandfathers did seldom or never. I was once in a conversation with a group of women when one woman said that her son-in-law was babysitting the kids. Several other women jumped in to say that he was not babysitting his own children; he was being their dad. I think the conversation moved on to consider whether gender identity and work roles—that divide according to gender—are determined and fixed by biology or, instead, determined by social environment and the way people are brought up.

My dad—actually my stepdad—and my brother Barry were raised in households where the daughters and sisters took charge of the caregiving. That's what happened when Mom got sick. The sisters took charge. Dad and Barry got a pass.

I hear many stories about men who care for their aging, Alzheimer's-stricken spouses who, when their wives are receiving care in a nursing home, visit them daily, feed them soup, and sing to them about the old days. I'd like to write about that happening in our family . . . it makes a good story . . . and I might be able to dig up a few pieces of supportive evidence to imply that scenario; however, the story would not match the reality of our situation.

Dad seldom visited Mom. His visits didn't decline over time as she lost memory of him. From the very first, he didn't visit much. We were saddened by the fact, but there was not much we could do about it. He was ready to do whatever—something, anything when a specific action was called for. We excused his hesitancy to see her—to just be with her—because his inaction could be explained in many ways. There was, of course, the grief at the loss of his wife to something so much beyond his control. That he was over ten years younger than she exacerbated the loss. He was still relatively youthful and his plans had included their continued travel and ardent support of the local sports teams. He was robbed of his golden years with his wife. And then there was the fact that in the years leading up to the eventual diagnosis of her illness, living with Mom had not been easy.

We wondered if she resented him because, at her age, she was now perceived as an old woman and he was not yet perceived as an old man. For whatever reason, she increasingly came to hold him in contempt. All five of us were uncomfortable around them because we knew that she could turn on him quickly. She seemed to reserve such anger for him—a hateful attitude that was never directed at anyone else. We can only imagine what happened when no one else was around. Everyone has faults, and my stepdad was not without a few, but even his gestures of kindness were rebuffed. There was no way for him to win. His mental state regarding the whole situation might best be described as one of confusion . . . that, and pain.

When we decided she needed professional care, he might have felt relief—not only to be free of the increasingly hostile behavior, but also relieved because he finally had an explanation for that behavior. At the time, however, we weren't thinking about him. She had told all of us separately and collectively that when she could no longer take care of herself, she didn't want to be left with *him*. A big part of the decision to move her to a care facility had been that we knew he would not do well as a caregiver. He was a military man, good at following orders and not so good at reading other people's needs—and especially the needs of his incapacitated and aging wife.

I remember when we devised a plan for helping him make Mom take her medicine. It was a great plan . . . right up to the time it failed. Mom resented Dad's reminding her to take her pills. We found a little platter and a bud vase, bought some medicine cups, and outlined how Dad would keep fresh flowers on hand so that he could present Mom her daily dosage. We sisters agreed this was an excellent plan. Unfortunately, Dad neglected the flowers and the little platter part and put the pills in the medicine cup and brusquely said, "Here." How foolish of us not to see that this plan wasn't going to work.

Once Mom was at the nursing home, he was attentive to all the tasks that needed his action. He needed to make sure that her phone was hooked up, a new TV was ready to go, the favorite chair from home was moved to the right spot, and she had the right kind of adult diapers, the ones that she could call panties. Just visiting—being with her—was too difficult. He required an action, a purpose.

Dad understood that he was needed to pay the bills or move a piece of furniture. But after Mother's connection to him faded from her mind, he no longer thought his presence was necessary. He seldom visited her, even when he went into the nursing home to pay her bill. He rationalized that she didn't know him anyway, but my sisters and I knew Mother's recognition of him was not the point. Mom lived in the moment, not in reality. We knew that we needed to be with her not because she remembered who we were, but because she needed to have someone in that room who remembered who she was.

Over the years, my brother's response to Mom's situation was similar to his dad's. He was always there to help with money for something she needed or to do what we sisters asked of him. Sometimes, I wonder if his gender-role preparation made him more like his dad than like his sisters . . . or is that innate male behavior? . . . or his individual personality? Trying to piece together this puzzle of how gender roles have played a part in Dad's and Barry's ability to be caregivers is a subject better left to sociologists or psychologists.

I need to stick to what I know firsthand. My brother, Mother's only son, was born when I was 14 years old. At 17, I no longer lived at home, so in the grand scheme of things, we had very little time to forge a strong sibling relationship. My early years were spent in a different household. The memories I have of Barry's formative years probably include events he either doesn't know or doesn't remember.

A couple of things I remember about his birth are vivid in my mind. One was that I was embarrassed by Mom's pregnancy. Yes, a foolish reaction, but at 14, the embarrassment was an intense burden. That it was unreasonable made it no less heavy. I also remember seeing the new baby boy for the first time. One of us three children from the first marriage described him as "wrinkled and squished." I have no memory of what he looked like, but I do remember the new father's reaction to the description. When he talked to Mom privately, he asked her if she thought Barry was OK. He was genuinely worried. I don't know how I know this information; perhaps I was told years later. And, of course, the perfect, fair-haired boy was OK. Why this event has stayed with me all these years, I believe, is because I was surprised to learn that the words of a 14-year-old child could have the power to worry adults.

Another memory is of Mother scrubbing the kitchen floor just days after Barry was born. I can picture her yet, and along comes the memory of my nonchalant reaction to it: Mom scrubbing the floor. What's new? It wasn't until after I had given birth to a perfect, fair-haired boy of my own that the realization struck me. I hadn't offered to help. I had not said, "Mom, get up. Go back to bed and rest. Let me finish this."

All this is to say I loved the little boy and love the adult person he became. We shared a mother's attention for a short time—and perhaps this woman, our mother, was a different person for each of us, considering her age, the differing situations, and new expectations. Yet our familial tie meant that I could read pain on his face the day when I knew he was the first family member Mom didn't recognize.

The sad event unfolded this way. I had returned home for a summer visit with Mom, and, as usual, my two sisters from the first family traveled there as well. We were taking her out to lunch. We fixed her hair, put some lipstick on her, and signed her out of the nursing home. Lori, the youngest sister, couldn't get away from work, but her young daughter joined us. Barry could break away from work long enough to be there.

He arrived just as we were ordering. Each of us stood to give him a hug as he sat down at the end of the table. Mom was in her wheelchair at the other end. She paid no attention to him. He said hi to her from a distance in an awkward and self-conscious way. I suspected she had failed to recognize him before this. Otherwise, he would have gone to Mother first. We chatted, and the conversation turned to our great-grandfather's home in the hills of Tennessee, a homestead preserved for family and remembered fondly by hundreds of Poag ancestors scattered across the country.

Mother was not speaking much by this time, but she could still follow a conversation. She entered the conversation by saying, "What does that man know about Pappy Poag?" She addressed the question to those of us near her and pointed her finger at Barry.

"Mom, I'm your son, Barry."

"Who?" She shook her head in disbelief and looked away, confused.

A heavy silence descended on all of us. One more loss in a long list of forgetting. And Barry was swallowed up by the swirling black hole of Alzheimer's disease, as if he were sinking from her view. The rest of us were there to watch all the versions of him as a child and as an adult—all the memories of his childhood, his boisterous laugh, his energetic spirit, and now this man with the pained face—sinking out of sight. All the rest of us followed into the swirl eventually.

Dad was next. Mom failed to recognize her husband soon after. It was their anniversary. She asked Lori about the man standing near them, and when Lori told her that was her husband, she replied, "I'm married?"

Alzheimer's disease erased from Mother's ailing brain the ability to recognize her son, her husband, and her daughters— the one who was with her most the last to be lost. If I ponder the order in which we disappeared, I tend to link her ability to hold onto memory of us to our physical presence during caregiving, but thinking about that serves no purpose. I can only assume that gender-role development that assigns caregiving tasks to women creates an especially difficult road for husbands and sons. Our family conditioned its daughters to *do something* even if it's wrong. In some ways, that's easier. Our family, and perhaps societal norms for Dad's and Barry's generations, made them bystanders, helpless to do anything other than stare directly into a problem that is difficult to face.

CHAPTER 20
ADJUSTING TO THE NEW NORMAL

When we are no longer able
to change a situation,
we are challenged to change ourselves.
~ VICTOR FRANKL

Life with Mom became one adjustment after another. Holidays always presented problems.

The year Mother fell into the Christmas tree, Lori decided she could no longer take Mom for an overnight stay. Mom was restricted to the main level of Lori's house because maneuvering the staircase was no longer possible. Even the ground level was difficult for her because the family room required one step down. When she misjudged that one step, the Christmas tree broke her fall. This was fortunate because she could have stumbled toward the fireplace. But the tree was obliterated—most of the ornaments crushed, the angel from the top flopping on the floor. My sister needed help lifting her from the debris. Later, having forgotten the incident, Mother sat on the sofa studying the lopsided tree. "That sure is a pitiful-looking Christmas tree!" Explanation would serve no purpose.

The next Christmas Lori took Mother to Barry's house for gift opening and then back to the nursing facility for the night. The gathering included Mom and Dad, Lori's family, Barry's family, as well as his wife's parents. I received the report of how Mother had sat silent and confused. I knew I had seen this re-action myself at other times when too many people were gath-ered with too much talking for her to sort out. Her presence at family gatherings moved from sad to sadder. She thought Barry, her only son, was her cousin, and she had no idea who Cindy's parents were. Having lost her ability to carry on a conversation, she spoke in one-sentence pronouncements, including tactlessly pointing out who was overweight.

My sister-in-law's parents tried to make the best of the situation. Finally they said, "Oh, I think you know us. Don't you, Jacque?" I imagined their words were delivered in the high-pitched voice often reserved for children. Cindy's parents are very nice people, but I couldn't help thinking, "OK, you folks can take a turn denying the severity of her disease, and we'll see how that works." I was moving past denial and adjusting to changes in mother's behavior. (Although, I perhaps needed to work on my flippant, sarcastic nature.)

I could no longer have the same comfortable relationship with Mother that I had developed throughout my lifetime. The new task of relating required a new way of looking at her altered personality. The old relationship was lost. Evidently, I needed to learn the lesson over and over again. Each reminder that I must not revert to my previous frame of reference was accompanied by a pain that never dulled.

I learned it again the year my mother ended a tradition I hadn't realized was important to me. One Christmas, Mother handed me a gift bag, saying, "This is just something I picked out for you. It's not your main gift." This was something special, an afterthought . . . a personal little something she had found at the last minute that reminded her of me. Having no time to wrap it up, she grabbed a previously used Christmas gift bag. The bag had contained last year's gift from me to her, so she had crossed out the names and labelled the bag from her to me. The next year I found the little bag in my saved Christmas wrappings and decided to give her an extra gift in the same bag. I crossed out the names and recorded the date. The following year I got the Christmas bag back, a personal and special gift inside for me with the date on the tag and names once again reversed. Thus the tradition began.

We looked for the bag under the tree each subsequent year. When she saw me place the familiar package under the tree, she would exclaim, "Oh, you brought the bag!" Our gift exchange continued for a few years after the onset of Alzheimer's disease and the yearly advance of its ravaging effects. Having watched her marked decline in one year, I knew our tradition would soon stop.

When that time arrived, it pained my heart to see her pick up the tattered bag and lay it aside, not recognizing the gift. I later rescued the bag from the discarded paper pile. It was old and needed to be thrown away, but with a sad heart I packed it away with the other Christmas trimmings. Families sometimes don't know what their traditions are until they lose them. The next Christmas I told a friend about finding the bag and how hard it was to begin the Christmas season without looking for a special gift for my Mom. My friend insisted I give a gift in the tattered Christmas bag. "You need to do this for you," she said. "Your mother has Alzheimer's. You don't!"

I needed to give the gift and claim the joy of giving, not expecting it to be returned and knowing I would once again need to rescue the bag from her pile of Christmas wrappings. I must do this because Mother could not. She could never go back to who she had been. The burden of adjustment falls to those who continue a relationship with the one who has Alzheimer's disease.

CHAPTER 21

THE RECIPE FOR CHOCOLATE GRAVY AND OTHER MYSTERIES

"It gets late early."
~YOGI BERRA

There is no "You Are Here" on the Alzheimer's progression chart. You just never know when your mother will mentally be there one day and then mysteriously gone the next. Her recall of events became less and less certain, but then she would rally to supply some unique detail from years long ago. The past soon faded as well. It was a herky-jerky decline toward forfeiting a life. And when memory is gone it always seems sudden.

I should have asked her about the things I needed to know. It's not as if I didn't know that the end of memory would come. I should have reckoned with this sad fact. When my grandfather died, I realized for the first time that I had neglected to ask about his life before it was too late. I was in my twenties and thought of my grandfather only in terms of his relationship to me, not as a man who was born in 1900. He was 14 years old at the beginning of World War I; I never thought about that. He was a farmer and then a businessman. I never asked what his life was like or how he made decisions. How did his family fare during the Great Depression? Where was he when Pearl Harbor was bombed? He could play the piano by ear, but did he ever study music? How did he meet my grandma?

And yet, I did the very same thing with my mother. I needed to know a hundred things—big and small. I needed to know her recipe for chocolate gravy. There were so many talks I postponed because the day's problems were sufficiently time consuming. Perhaps I refused to think about her inevitable death. I wished for the final stage to be far away and believed it so. As the family identified Mom's behaviors, we couldn't place her at, say, five or seven years out from the end point when she would forget how to swallow and starve her own body.

Even when a family knows all of these things, most families don't know exactly when the Alzheimer's countdown clock started. Our family identified when the signs of the disease began long after the fact. Looking back, we put the pieces together.

For one thing, hiding that something is wrong is common when people have Alzheimer's disease. Most families discover that Mom and Dad protect each other. They finish each other's sentences. They fill in the gaps of memory easily and seamlessly. No cause for alarm. Also, there is the effort to hide embarrassment for the spouse when she does such silly things. Leaving her purse, forgetting an appointment, not finding the right words. Then there is the hope that the medications may be working. Maybe there will be more time after all. It's hard to know how far or at what speed the disease might have progressed without treatment. All of these factors make it difficult for the family to see the progression of the disease in one individual case.

But in the end, with the current state of treatment, the family who does not ask the right questions or who does not pay attention to expressed history will lose important details, not only personal histories and medical histories, but also cultural traditions—like the recipe for chocolate gravy.

Finding a recipe that matches how Mom made chocolate gravy is not something easy to do, even with Google. I found out that this chocolatey sauce, which is served for breakfast over buttermilk biscuits, is a Southern dish. My granny made it as a treat for my sisters and me and Mother made it after that. Perhaps it was a reward for good behavior or good grades, but I always felt it was a reward for being me—loved unconditionally and deserving of good things.

I've found recipes but not the right one. I've tried to create the taste with multiple experiments, some rendering a gritty texture and others closely resembling pudding. Perhaps it could be true that you can't go back again. The memory of the thing in the past will remain better, bigger, richer. Still, the recipe for chocolate gravy is a real thing, a piece of family identity that, for reasons I do not fully understand, is important to me. Its absence feels like loss.

What I have been able to discover of our family history is that we are "next-year people." My maternal grandparents moved to California from the South during the 50s. I vaguely connected the reason for the move to the dust bowl, but the timing is 20 years off. Perhaps they were just slow to give up. They had been farmers and thus earned the descriptor "next year" people, those who are always looking ahead to next year when they again go up against Mother Nature and literally bet the farm on it. My paternal grandparents stayed put in the rich Arkansas farmlands just west of the Mississippi River. They were next-year people, too.

So, I guess I am next-year people as well, and I will keep searching and experimenting until, by God, I have that recipe for chocolate gravy, made the way my mother did and serve it over buttermilk biscuits for breakfast. It's a perfectly horrible dish—so very bad for a person's health, but so perfectly good for a person's soul.

CHAPTER 22

MOM AND ALICE

> You have forgotten who you are and so have
> forgotten me. Look inside yourself, Simba.
> You are more than what you have become. You
> must take your place in the Circle of Life.
> ~ MUFASA'S GHOST IN *THE LION KING*

As Mother's memory was slipping so surely away, I continually faced the pain I felt each time she could not call me by name. More and more she was losing ability to recognize her children. I remembered with panic the time my good friend showed up on my doorstep the day her mother with Alzheimer's disease had not recognized her for the first time. She couldn't get the words out before she started to cry. Each time I left Mother was difficult because I never knew whether she would know me the next time I came.

Seeing my new baby granddaughter was always joyous after leaving Mom. I think Alice was about 10 months old when I had a chance to visit the baby girl. I hadn't seen Alice in a couple of months, and since babies change so fast, I wondered if she would know me. As I entered the room, I saw a sudden flash of recognition in Alice's eyes. She, as yet, had no vocabulary to access. She could not yet run to me with outstretched arms shouting, "Grandma, Grandma!" But there it was—a look that made her light up. Her eyes said, "I don't know your name, but I know you are mine. I know you are important to me. You belong to me and I belong to you. I'm so glad you're here. Please stay awhile."

My epiphany was this. I had seen that same flash of recognition in my mother's eyes the day before. She no longer knew my name, but she knew that I belonged to her and she belonged to me. Now I knew that Great Granddaughter and Great Grandmother had this in common, even though the trajectory of their lives pointed in opposite directions. If their lives were charted on a line graph, one line would show a promising incline; the other, a depressing decline. Yet, in this moment, for me and perhaps in me, their lives intersected.

As Mom was slowly losing language, I discovered that Alzheimer's cannot take away one thing: love, pure and simple. Even after Mom had no flash of recognition when I walked into the room—even after she might politely thank me for delivering her towels as if I were the nurse's aide—I held on to this shared but unspoken knowledge that I belonged to her and she belonged to me. Not Alzheimer's, and not even death, can change that. And now this new revelation: the sense of belonging lives on in the baby girl. Affirmation of the circle of life is enough to sustain me.

CHAPTER 23

THE POWER OF MUSIC

> Where words fail, music speaks.
> ~ HANS CHRISTIAN ANDERSON

I recall Mother singing with my sisters and me when we were very young. She couldn't carry a tune in a bucket. After Mom and Dad had been retired for a few years and when the signs of Alzheimer's disease were just becoming apparent, Dad talked about her singing in the car all the way back from a trip to Branson, Missouri. He said he was shocked there were so many verses to "America the Beautiful." She knew several and repeated them many times for hundreds of miles. He did not interrupt her, preferring to stay silent—at that point he was walking on eggshells. That, and he was career military, so there was the patriotic element. He told us the story with a mixed tone of sadness and humor, hesitating with a long pause and then saying, "You know, your mom doesn't sing well."

Once an apparently tone-deaf man who sat near her in church told her she had a lovely voice. From then on, she decided not to worry about how she sounded. She belted out hymns, making a joyful noise, to the end of her church-going days. Even after she was in the nursing home and someone had to get her ready and take her to church, she sang proudly with the congregation. Even after the names of her children had slipped away from her, she sang out, and the strangest thing was that she remembered the words to her favorite old hymns. How could it be that she could remember all the words to "Amazing Grace" yet not remember my name?

After completing a layperson's survey of research on the subject—which means I consulted Internet sources and checked a couple of journals at a good library—I've come up with an explanation that makes sense to me. I know attempting to explain a complex idea in simple terms always risks distortion by oversimplification, but here, I am attempting to arrive at an analysis of music and memory so that I might answer my question. Even though the explanation is not simple, here is what I've learned.

The brain handles music-related memory in interesting and complex ways. Much of what researchers know about the brain's ability to process music and memory of music results from use of functional magnetic resonance imaging. Those who study the perception of music have learned music touches many areas of the brain (Suomen, 2011). Researchers look at not only where music memory is stored, but also how it got there and how it is retrieved. In addition to believing that music information is stored in multiple areas of the brain, they also believe it got there in multiple ways (Ashford, 2010). All of these complexities must be accounted for if I am to answer my question about Mom's memory and why her diseased brain could not retrieve information about me.

In order to explain, I need to talk about two types of memory: explicit memory and implicit memory. Explicit memory is conscious recollection. Implicit memory is unconscious, sometimes unintentional, memory.

I want to concentrate on one subcategory of explicit memory called episodic memory. Episodic memory is the first key term of two I want the reader to understand. The second key term is procedural memory—another way of saying implicit memory. I want to use the term procedural memory because it is a better descriptor of the process I want to describe. Knowing about epi-sodic memory will explain why my mother did not know my name, and knowing about procedural memory will explain why she remembered hymns. The following answers the question, "How does that happen?"

Episodic memory is about autobiography—stuff that deals with the events of a person's life (Mastin, 2010a). Episodic memory is the kind of explicit memory that would allow my mother to know that I am her daughter because when the brain is working properly, this kind of memory enables people to ac-cess contextual clues—the times, the places, the events . . . the episodes that comprise their lives.

In addition to episodic memory—the one important in this discussion—there is another kind of memory in the category of explicit memory: semantic memory. I'll briefly define it be-cause people often better understand a complex idea like epi-sodic memory by knowing what it is not. Semantic memory is memory of things learned on purpose but which are not directly related to identity and life story (Mastin, 2010b). It includes re-membering the capital of Peru, the multiplication tables, or the historical difference between the United Nations and the League of Nations. In other words, abstract knowledge.

Several years after the onset of Alzheimer's disease, Mother lost explicit memory, both semantic and episodic. She did not remember that Lima is the capital of Peru, and neither did she remember my name. I was lost to my mother long before I lost her. Yet my mother remembered hymns. That is because her fa-vorite hymns were not stored in episodic or semantic memory. They were stored in procedural memory, which saves informa-tion regarding how to do something without thinking about it (Mastin, 2010a). Driving a car, making a bed, and playing a mu-sical instrument are examples. These things are learned through repeated practice until they become automatic. People might know the experience of leaving work for home, intending to go to the grocery store first, but ending up in their driveway because the conscious mind was still working on some problem of the day while the unconscious mind—the procedural memory—was remembering every turn needed to get home.

Another example of using procedural memory is the ability to write easily with the dominant hand. This is an activity practiced so many times that it becomes easy. Switching to the left hand—or the right, if you're left-handed—is difficult. It takes concentration because people have to consciously think about it. Writing with the non-dominant hand is an unrehearsed skill requiring a higher level of cognitive functioning. Any skill repeatedly practiced and stored through procedural memory becomes automatic.

Mother acquired the ability to write easily with her right hand by repeated practice. Her memory of hymns was acquired in exactly the same way, by years of singing the hymns over and over again. Each was stored as procedural memory. Researchers say that the damaging effects of Alzheimer's disease spares procedural memory that has been well rehearsed and disrupts retrieval of episodic memory, the autobiographical kind—the personal or emotional recollections specific to a context, time, and place (Golby et al., 2005). It's like saying that Mother's procedural memory was stored on a lower, reachable shelf. Episodic memory, in contrast, was not rehearsed—not automatic—and was stored via more complex cognitive functions related to the events—the episodes—of her life. It is as if these episodic memories were not only stored on a higher shelf but also as if they were packaged in millions of boxes labelled The Time I Took My Children to Summer Camp or How I Felt While Playing Basketball in High School or Why My First Marriage Failed. Those boxes are harder to reach; they are also tougher to unpack.

My mother never worked at memorizing the names of her children. We were not people whose names had to be rehearsed like the recitation of the months of the year. My mother did not store the names of her children in the same place in her brain where she stored unconscious, procedural memory that she used to recall her favorite hymns. Mom's children were not abstractions to her. We existed for her in real time and space—in real episodes that made up her life. In her mind, knowing our names was tied to the people she experienced, operating in specific contextual circumstances, and stored in her episodic memory.

Since episodic memory is exactly the kind of memory that is most damaged by Alzheimer's disease, Mother could no longer access memories that contained my name and other information that would allow her to recognize me. Neural pathways in my mothers's brain were obstructed by plaques and tangles, while the procedural memory of hymns, committed to memory early and purposefully repeated, were spared and readily available to her long after onset of the disease. Figuring out these facts made Mom's condition easier to understand, but no easier to endure.

Is there any good news we can take from this sad lesson? Researchers believe that when dementia patients can no longer access memories of their lives packed away deep in their episodic memory, music of their past may have the ability to activate memories not accessible by visual cues or spoken prompts (Bergland, 2013).

That makes sense to me. Music touches every aspect of our lives, affecting us emotionally, physically, spiritually, and aesthetically. Music is important to human beings—even, it seems, when we produce it badly or understand its structure minimally. The link between music and memory has always seemed magical. Even children—perhaps especially children—know its power. The way we learn the alphabet is by singing it. Rhythm and rhyme and alliteration help us learn and remember many things: the number of days in each month ("Thirty days hath September, April, June . . .") or how a bill is passed (the Schoolhouse Rock history song). Information set to music is easier to remember. If we are asked to repeat the words to "Take Me Out to the Ball

Game," we are most successful if we sing them rather than say them—or at least recall the melody in our heads.

Pre-literate societies used chanting, alliteration, rhythm, and rhyme to recall huge amounts of information. *The Iliad, The Odyssey,* and *Beowulf* were memorized pieces of literature. In fact, beginning pieces of literature for most great cultures were poems because poetry provided the musical devices that promoted memorization and thus preserved the information before things were written down.

Victor Hugo said that music expresses that which cannot be put into words and that which cannot remain silent. All cultures create music. We should not underestimate the role of music in human culture. Music memories are special. Pieces of our lives that we associate with music fit into numerous categories. Perhaps it's not surprising that those who study the brain have found music memories stored in so many areas. To return to my previous analogy, music memories seem to be stored on various shelves and in many separate boxes. This might also explain why the power of music is such that when we hear a certain song from long ago, we can recall where we were, what we were wearing, and how we felt when the song was playing in the background. Apparently those music memories, stored on many shelves and in many boxes, are cross-referenced and continually updated and reclassified.

Of course, the file-system comparison is an overly-simplified conceptualization. Science-y people, like my daughter and her friends, would say the analogy is too narrow. They might say a better comparison would be a web . . . like a spider web . . . or the Internet. One strand of thought connects to another so nothing is in just one place.

Researchers have determined a profound connection between music and otherwise unreachable memories in geriatric patients (Hsu, 2009). Providing a dementia patient with a well-known song specifically from his or her past supplies the context—the time and place—that can trigger episodic memory, the auto-biographical memory. Not just any music will do. Music most likely to awaken memories is the music from adolescence and young adulthood.

According to Levitin (2007), "We tend to remember things that have an emotional component because our amygdala and neurotransmitters act in concert to 'tag' the memories as some-thing important" (p. 231). Emotionally charged information about events from formative years is stored in many categories in the brain. Often memories are connected to music, and when songs of the time period are available to dementia patients, the music facilitates retrieval of information. They are able to recall who they were, where they were, and how they felt when they first heard Benny Goodman play "In the Mood" or the time they sang along to Bing Crosby's "I'll Be Seeing You." For those not in my mother's generation, a different list of songs would retrieve memory.

Music therapists, geriatric caregivers, and others who deal with elderly patients have begun to tap the power of music for treatment of dementia. One organization, Music & Memory, has achieved success in the practical application of music (ABC News, 2014).

This group delivers iPods to patients with Alzheimer's and other forms of dementia. The iPods have playlists specific to the music of each patient's youth. As a result, the patients are given a link to their past. Because of music's ability to trigger memory connected to familiar songs, families and caregivers note im-provement in patients' abilities to converse and stay present in the moment. Music has the power to bring the patient "back to life." In fact, after repeated periods of time in which patients experience the music that was important to them, they achieved higher scores in tests of cognitive ability (Sample, 2013).

Another organization, the Giving Voice Initiative based in Minneapolis/St. Paul, is aware of the research that shows memories and emotions are stimulated during music activities. This non-profit organization operates the Giving Voice Chorus, a music community of people with dementia and their care partners who prepare for public musical performances guided by specially trained music professionals. This community has expanded to establish multiple choirs, all of which allow singers to significantly improve quality of life. The experience provides purpose and camaraderie by participation in music, through which choir members access the parts of the brain where knowledge and skill are the last to be affected by Alzheimer's disease (Huppert, 2014).

Music sticks with people. Once, after Mother was first in the nursing care facility, I took her to a musical presentation in the large gathering room of the home. She was still ambulatory at the time, but many patients were rolled in by nurses pushing their wheelchairs. I noticed a woman who was totally disengaged—slumped in her chair, motionless and emotionless. Fearing the time when Mom would get to that stage, I noticed the woman was tapping her foot to the beat of the music. I pointed it out to one of the nurses who was busy transporting patients. "Yes," she told me quickly, "I guess she played in her family's band."

Music therapists say music can reduce wandering, restlessness, and agitated behaviors in dementia patients, as well as improve cognitive function (Clair, 2016). There are a number of explanations for how these improvements happen. One is that dementia patients feel bombarded with large amounts of random and confusing input and have difficulty sorting it out. They perceive familiar music as organized sound (patterned, sequenced, repeated) that buffers the confusing noise in their surroundings. The improvements in behaviors are significant when added to the improved social interaction that occurs when patients are "brought back to life" as familiar music triggers memories of important personal events in their autobiographical past. At the very least, music therapy provides the added benefit of exercise because individuals retain the ability to move to a rhythm even in advanced stages of the disease (Schaeffer, 2016).

The movie *The Shawshank Redemption* has a great scene in which a prison yard full of tough and often belligerent men stop suddenly to listen to an aria from Mozart's *Marriage of Figaro* when the main character, Andy, boldly broadcasts it over the intercom. The men are enthralled, transported by clear, sweet, and melancholy voices singing in a language the men do not understand. Another main character, Red, describes the music this way:

> I have no idea what those two Italian ladies were singing about. Truth is, I don't want to know. Some things are best left unsaid. I'd like to think they were singing about something so beautiful, it can't be expressed in words, and makes your heart ache because of it. I tell you, those voices soared higher and farther than anybody in a gray place dares to dream. It was like some beautiful bird flapped into our drab little cage and made those walls dissolve away, and for the briefest of moments, every last man in Shawshank felt free (Darabont, 1994).

When my daughter went to college, we sent her off as a piano major and she came back to us a scientist. When she got married, I was not surprised she cared little about the flowers, but the music was extremely important to her. She called to ask about which songs her grandmother would recognize. Her background in music and her study of the brain told her she needed just the right song when Grandma walked down the aisle at the wedding.

We do not know if Grandma recognized the music specifically chosen for her that day. Neither do we know if she was freed from her imprisonment as she was escorted to a seat up front. Perhaps the magic of music unlocked from her memory the words to the song she heard the string quartet play. Perhaps she remembered the words to the favorite hymn because the lyrics, having been sung so many times, were stored in procedural memory. Perhaps, also, the music that had been part of the soundtrack of her life released from episodic memory details of her life and her place within the life of her family gathered for the wedding. I know I can repeat all the words to that song because the melody is firmly stuck in my head.

CHAPTER 24

HAPPINESS IS SOMETHING YOU DECIDE AHEAD OF TIME

> Happiness is a choice that
> requires effort at times.
> ~ AESCHYLUS

As Mother's disease progressed, my anxiety level increased each time I entered the nursing home to see her. Since she seldom recognized me anymore, I developed the habit of announcing who I was when I entered her room to avoid her look of confusion. I was protecting myself more than I was seeking to lessen her bewilderment. Sometimes it worked. She had not forgotten that a daughter is someone she was supposed to love.

"Hi, Mom, it's your oldest and favorite daughter!"

"That's what you think," she once replied with a smile. She was having a good day.

Whenever I returned to town to see Mom, my sisters generally arrived from near and far. With each visit we were becoming less distinct to her. She had not called us by name for quite some time, but she knew we were her daughters collectively, though not specifically as individuals. Her characteristic teasing and sense of humor served her well in hiding how much she was or was not perceiving.

On one visit when I was there for about three weeks—seeing her all day almost every day—I took her down to the Side Board, a little cafe for residents and visitors. I stepped away to get my coffee and her hot chocolate. As I returned to our table and set down the mugs, she looked at me with delighted surprise and called me by name. "Regina, I'm so glad you are here!" Clearly, she knew exactly who I was as well as my relationship to her. It was the only time during the three-week trip I had all of her back for a brief few minutes.

On the last day of that extended visit, she gave me an odd and precious gift. Repeatedly during my time there, she had asked, "What are we doing here?" This was not a complaint; we had already passed her complaint and anger stage. Her simple request for information still had power to sting because it required telling her that this was where she lived now—all the more difficult because I wondered if she remembered she had a spacious home only miles away. Most often my answer was a diversion of sorts. But this time I answered her by saying, "Mom, you're old. You can't remember things."

"Oh." Her response was a whisper.

So I continued. "Mom, you are safe. You are cared for here. If you can't be happy, at least be content because you are OK."

"All right. I'll just go for happy."

A precious gift!

CHAPTER 25

USEFUL THINGS WE HAVE LEARNED

> "It is the obvious that is so difficult
> to see sometimes. People say,
> 'It's as plain as the nose on your face.' But
> how much of the nose on your face
> can you see, unless someone
> holds a mirror up to you?"
> ~ Isaac Asimov, *I, Robot*

Somewhere along the way in our family's journey, we stopped trying to understand why Mom had been burdened with Alzheimer's disease. We moved past the impossible task of trying to make Mom better. Just as she decided to be happy, we decided to be content. Settling for contentment freed us from being overwhelmed by emotion, guilt, and sorrow so that we could do what needed to be done. We asked, "What are the requirements of the moment?" Looking back, we realize we learned many things that may be useful to others.

One of the things we learned in the early stages of the disease was to limit Mom's choices. We noticed that she never seemed to be hungry enough to order anything at a restaurant, but she would surely eat whatever we had ordered for ourselves. We finally realized that menus had become difficult for her to decipher. Too many choices. We began pointing out two or three items we knew she would like. "Mom, the BLT is here and the grilled chicken salad is here." She happily accepted one of our suggestions, and everyone was able to enjoy lunch.

The move to offering fewer options was the same one we had used with our children. Saying "You can play in the front yard or the backyard" limited their choices to acceptable locations. Later, of course, they would learn to ask about playing at the playground or at Anne's or Shawn's house. Developmental stages shift with growing children just as they shift with declining parents.

The needs of children continually change as they grow up. How to deal with a crying four-year-old is different from how to deal with a crying fourteen-year-old. And just when you figure out how to address the daughter who is crying because some of her friends have already been asked to the ninth grade dance and she hasn't, you blink twice and then you listen to her frantic cry on the phone because bad weather caused her to miss the plane to Atlanta to defend her doctoral dissertation. How to deal with a mom in the early stages of AD is also different from how to deal with her in the later stages. Too soon, giving Mom three choices at the restaurant became giving two choices, then one, and finally the discovery that it was just easier to order something for her.

Along with learning that Mom could better handle a limited range of choices, we also learned to avoid noise clutter. As her condition worsened, she was less able to filter aural stimulation. We learned that having the TV going and three of us talking in what seemed to us a rapid but reasonable conversation was too stressful for her. Saying "Mom, Mom, Mom" did not get her attention; it created noise. We worked to eliminate background noise, limit speakers in the conversation, slow down, and speak short sentences in quiet tones. Loudly repeating words she didn't seem to understand didn't help. Volume was not the problem.

Her brain's ability to decipher what the words meant was the problem.

We came to understand the importance of listening for the intent of her often anxious words, as well as watching her body language. Once we identified the need, we adjusted to address that need with a statement, repeating back what we observed and thus avoiding a question that would require her to formulate an answer. For example, we said, "You need a tissue for your running nose, don't you?" rather than "What do you need?"

Agitation when there was no obvious reason might have meant that she needed to go to the bathroom or any number of other things. We wondered at the endless frustration a caregiver must feel when she has sole responsibility for a person with dementia. The caregiver must continually figure out what the patient needs. Sometimes it was hard to tell the difference between pain, discontent or anxiety. Trying to be a mind reader of a diseased mind is tough work. No doubt this is the reason so many experts emphasize the importance of caregivers having breaks from the tiring routine. They must remember to take care of themselves as well as the patient.

When prompting Mother to do something, we learned we should not explain why. Defending rationale is a customary thing in our family, but when Mother's communication skills failed, talking about why an action was necessary became a waste of time for us and a source of frustration for her. It wasn't as if Mom was going to determine her own course of action or dazzle us with a superior contradictory plan. Comprehending what we wanted her to do was all she could handle. Instead of saying, "The restaurant may be a little chilly this time of year. Do you think you're are going to need your sweater?" We learned to say, "Here's your sweater." She was no longer capable of anticipating that a restaurant might be cool or figuring out that having a sweater would address the problem.

Later, she was no longer able to put on the sweater without prompting. Then we squeezed her arm gently and said, "Lift this arm," and that action would start the process. Sometimes using visual cues—using an action along with or instead of words—worked well. Wiping an imaginary crumb from the front of my shirt prompted the same motion for the real crumbs on her shirt. Clear, simple instruction in small steps worked best. Later yet, her mind couldn't recall the process for putting on the sweater, and we needed to lift her arm and put the sweater on her.

Taking her arm or hand and holding it firmly was welcome touch as long as it was not sudden. Since peripheral vision declines with age, it was important not to sneak up on her or make a sudden gesture to straighten her glasses, for example. I tried applying gentle pressure to the palm of her hand because I had heard this action would relieve stress and anxiety. Gentle touch could help her feel less anxious.

Sometimes it was difficult to understand that Mom was not being stubborn on purpose—Mom would have said "ornery." She had lost skills; she had lost memory of process. She could not decipher what was being said in a conversation, even though her hearing was good. She could no longer comprehend the organization of printed text, even though she could still read all of the words aloud. She could not manage the process of getting dressed, even though she was cold and needed the sweater in her lap. We needed to remember she was not trying to be difficult.

We always came back to communication as a sign of how bad off Mother really was. More and more as she struggled to find words, Mother pointed and shook her head as she tried to construct her thoughts. Clearly, she intended something; some thought was formed in her head that she could not convey through words. We learned to read her gestures rather than directing all our attention to deciphering her speech—which, at times, was an absurd combination of words. One time, I saw her shake her head in frustration and almost laugh at the disjointed phrase she had spoken. I think she was trying to point out that a squirrel had climbed the bird feeder just outside her window. Instead of saying, "See the squirrel," she said, "Western. It's the western." It must have been hard for her to have the thought right there in on the tip of her tongue and yet be unable to communicate it. We learned to listen to what she meant, not what she said.

We kept learning new things as Mom's condition worsened. I recall the time we learned that dementia patients may not remember new information . . . but they remember how they feel about it. At this point in the advance of the disease, Mom was unable to recall events from short-term memory, and I doubt she could have recited the names of my children without prompting.

While I was visiting Mom once, my son was admitted to the hospital with a medical emergency. All the family was worried about him. His dad was with him, and I was preparing to make the trip of several hundred miles to join them. Mother was distraught and urgent in her inquiry when I said good-bye to her. "Is there something wrong? Is there something wrong with Keith?" she asked. Even though she could not recount one detail of the previous evening's bad news, something in her brain was able to access the emotion attached to the news. She was able to pull that emotion from the clutter of details she could not seem to hold in her mind's grasp.

Since that time, I've read that caregivers report their loved ones seem upset for no apparent reason or act irrationally or show unexplained resentment. It seems that Alzheimer's patients can hold onto feelings they cannot explain for quite some time. This happens at the same time they are becoming less able to regulate emotion or work out the problem from which the emotion arises. Emotions, evidently, are harder to forget than facts.

Trying to explain to Mother why some petty grievance was not worth thinking about was probably more frustrating to her than to us. The part of her brain that could analyze the problem was no longer working. She was not thinking about the facts of the case. What she was holding onto was the emotional residue of those facts. The best response was to react to the emotion and feel bad that someone or something had upset her.

I have a friend whose mother was also afflicted with Alzheimer's disease, and we figured her mother's progression into the disease was about four years beyond Mother's stage. My friend shared that the family discovered their mother never seemed to have enough underwear. It was mysteriously disappearing. The problem was solved one day when she learned her mother was wearing every pair of panties she owned. Evidently, she recalled needing to do something about undergarments as part of good hygiene, but she failed to figure out the steps of the process for accomplishing her task. Mother exhibited similar odd behaviors. There always seemed to be some new evidence of the severity of the disease.

The learning curve is steep. Time is not your friend. Shifts happen.

As our family struggled to understand the behaviors associated with Mom's illness, we became aware of other people's perceptions of Mom's actions. One time, Mother went into a patient's room at the nursing home and turned off her oxygen because it was too noisy. Fortunately, an alarm signaled for help at the nurses' station. When we were told of Mother's action, we felt as if we had been called to school for a child's misbehavior. Of course we understood the severity of Mother's action and the concern expressed by the lady's family. Yet we also, for the first time, understood how sympathy is not evenly distributed.

The lady on oxygen was obviously sick, but Mother's sickness was not easy to see. If Mother's brain had been well, she would not have committed the crime. She was, however, no less deserving of compassion. People are apt to expect more of someone who does not look or sound sick. Strangely, when Mother's ability to communicate declined, people showed more compassion for the behaviors through which her disease was manifest because now her illness was apparent. If she sounded sick, it was easier to accept that she was sick. If people have cancer, everyone knows something bad has happened to them, but if people have schizophrenia, for example, some think they are at fault for behaviors they exhibit. There is a prevalent attitude that patients with mental illnesses have brought it on themselves. Both AD and schizophrenia are diseases of the brain. Our family learned that people in early stages of Alzheimer's disease are sometimes judged harshly for their behaviors, probably because their behaviors are sometimes embarrassing. Our mother was no less sick than the woman on oxygen.

By the end, we learned that we could do things we never thought we could do. Once, I asked Mom to give me her lower dentures. I rinsed them in hot water at the beverage area of the nursing home café, dried them off, and returned them to her. My granddaughters, Abigail Mae and Taylor Jane, looked at me with surprise and disgust. "Eeewww! Grandma, what are you doing?" they shrieked, as they looked around to see who was watching. I realized how nonchalant I had become when dealing with these everyday tasks. She was having trouble with her teeth, flipping them up with her tongue and cleaning her lower gums out with her finger. It was annoying, and she needed help.

There was a time early on when I couldn't have asked her to hand me her teeth, or spit food into my hand, or lift her feet so I could take her wet panties off. Learning that you can do what needs to be done is a valuable lesson. And whether or not you *want* to perform that difficult thing has nothing to do with the ability to do it.

My daughter Jill always comforted Mom with a matter-of-fact calmness that I admired. Her years as an RN taking care of others' needs served her well when dealing with her grandma. I was reminded of a few years earlier when Jill had helped during the final days of her other grandmother's fight with cancer. She had been there ready and more than able to provide bedside care for uncomfortable details that needed to be done. But I remember her saying, "I'm glad to help Grandma, but right now, I only want to be the granddaughter." Necessity makes us do things we might not have thought possible—things we never wanted to be responsible for doing.

Family members of some Alzheimer's patients say that their loved ones see themselves in mirrors and become alarmed by the intruder—a strange old woman in the room. As a result, families or nursing homes sometimes cover mirrors. Mother seemed perpetually surprised by her reflection and often reacted with a startled sigh that I interpreted as "What in the heck happened here?" Most of the time, she seemed to know she was looking at herself.

Except for one time. Mom and I were in a bathroom in the nursing home when Mom noticed herself in a full-length mirror. "Hi," she said and smiled at her reflection. It took me a minute to realize what was happening. Mom thought some other person was at the door. She leaned in to touch her head to the person in the mirror, as she often did when someone very near her smiled. Then she motioned to the woman, whispering with eyebrows raised, "Do you want to come in?" How curious that she couldn't recognize she was looking at herself. But she wasn't frightened. Usually, she was merely shocked by her age. On this occasion, she did not recognize herself in the present.

At times, Mother seemed to retreat into the past. Perhaps she felt safer there than in the unpredictable present. At first, we thought our job was to bring her back to the present—and thus keep her with us. But later, we realized our best and kindest choice was to meet her where she was. Our efforts to correct and contradict her were not going to alter the progression of the disease. Arguing about things brought her back to her cruel reality. We found it better to protect her by playing along. Talking about Jason and Angie's wedding as if it were yesterday or about

Keith swimming across the lake at the family reunion long ago was a much better reality.

Of all the things we learned, the most difficult lesson was the absolute absurdity of asking, "Don't you remember?" or "Mom, we told you about this yesterday." No, she was not going to remember. We had to keep learning it. She would not remember if she had eaten; she would not remember how old she was; she would not remember us.

Her granddaughter Justine was 23 the first time Grandma didn't know her. She was in the room at the nursing home when aides brought Mom back from an activity. "Grandma looked right through me," Justine told us later. "I could have been just anyone." Her eyes filled with tears. I realized she had made the difficult move from being a beloved granddaughter to being the functioning adult in the room. While Justine straightened her grandma's room and tried to talk with her, Grandma ignored her and seemed somewhat bothered by her presence. Her darling granddaughter was "just anyone."

Later that evening, Pam and I went to the nursing home to tuck Mom in and say good-bye before we left town. I had hoped that Justine would go along with us—it probably would have been good for her to see that Grandma didn't recognize us either. But it was getting late, and she had to work early the next morning. Once there, we busied ourselves getting Mom ready for bed, trying to say things that might identify us in her mind. We pointed to pictures of ourselves in much younger versions. Whatever our strategy on that evening, we nudged Grandma to the point of at least knowing we belonged to her and that she was in good hands.

As we tucked her in and said, "I love you," she tried to speak. The words would not come. But she vocalized something as she pointed at each of us and then rounded us up with a circular motion of her hand and put her hand to her heart. I answered her gesture by saying, "I know, Mom. You love us too." Love remains the shining light in a very dark place. I want to believe that "I love you" does not fail to connect on some level—no matter the stage of decline.

Over the years, we learned all the stages of the decline associated with Alzheimer's disease. We watched her function normally with occasional lapses in memory in the early stage. She forgot familiar words or the location of objects. When she moved into the second stage, mild cognitive decline, her difficulties became noticeable, but she was still functioning independently. At moderate cognitive decline, we saw problems in performing complex tasks, like keeping her checkbook straight or planning and preparing meals. In the moderately severe stage, she needed help with day-to-day activities, but she was able to feed and wash herself. She knew her family and the significant things about them even if she was foggy on details in short-term memory.

It wasn't until she declined to the severe stage that she could not remember significant details of her personal history or her family. Her personality changed, but only slightly, which is not always the case. She needed help with bathing, dressing, and feeding. Some patients at this stage exhibit compulsive, repetitive behaviors and the tendency to wander, but that was not the case with our mother. At the very severe or late stage, she lost the ability to interact with the environment. In her last few days, she could not hold her head erect. She no longer smiled.

Any good pamphlet on the disease could have informed us of the stages through which our mother would pass. But it was not until we watched her go through each of them that the stages became a lived experience—real rather than academic. A pamphlet is about someone else's mother . . . or father . . . or husband . . . or wife. The descriptions of the stages of Alzheimer's disease are words on a page until it's your mother.

All the things we learned are easy to describe now. They were not so easy to see when we were in the thick it . . . when the slow-motion journey of our mother was progressing to its inevitable conclusion. Some of the time, we were able to meet the challenges with kindness, skill, and humor. But most of the time, each as us wanted to fall to our knees and say, "Jesus, help me. I'm drowning here."

CHAPTER 26

MYSTIC CHORDS OF MEMORY

> I stood still, vision blurring,
> and in that moment,
> I heard my heart break. It was
> a small, clean sound,
> like the snapping of a flower's stem.
> ~ DIANA GABALDON, *DRAGONFLY IN AMBER*

We sat in the garden of the nursing home for a good portion of the afternoon, swaying back and forth in a bench-style gliding rocker. Having lost ability to form complete sentences for whatever thoughts she might have had, Mother pointed to the birds twittering in the trees or to the lush foliage and colorful array of flowers. I completed her thoughts with words I guessed she intended.

She was willing to struggle. "That . . . see . . . pretty . . . "

"Yes, the flowers are beautiful. These remind me of the tiger lilies along the fence posts on the way to Pappy Poag's house." I talked about her grandfather's house, secluded peacefully in the hills of Tennessee and still accessible if one is willing to cross two creeks. I talked about how she always said all the kids and grandkids loved to play in those creeks. Her eyes squinted; her brow furrowed. She was trying to remember and I thought she could almost grab the memory. It appeared to be right there within reach. Then it was gone and she returned to pointing to the flowers.

"Aren't these . . . nice . . . mmm . . . " She shook her head for lack of words.

I returned again and again to subjects of the distant past, weaving in thoughts about family members and happy times. The breeze was surprisingly cool for the middle of the summer.

"I think . . . I . . . know . . . uh . . . know . . . " Again she pointed to the pretty flowers while patting my knee affectionately with her other hand. She knew I was family, someone emerged from her blurry and ineffable past. She listened with interest and I imagined her struggling to drag a memory into the present. Then, with some urgency, she needed to go.

"Do you think it's time we headed back inside?" I asked.

She shook her head yes. I helped her back into the wheelchair and asked if we should stroll around the garden one more time, but she was very determined to go inside. As I took her to the room, she flagged down a passing nurse's aide. "I need to . . . have you . . . " The aide looked to me for a clue, but I didn't know what Mother needed. The nurse offered to bring fresh ice water to the room. She rushed off down the hall to get water; hers was as good a guess as any.

Next Mother stopped a cleaning lady and asked her, "Have you seen . . . ?" But the housekeeper had been busy and hadn't seen anyone or anything. As Mother became more anxious, she stopped everyone we passed, often grabbing an arm or hand. "Have you . . . have you seen . . . my . . . "

She stopped other people's children, children whose mothers had more feeble bodies than hers, but far clearer minds. "Have you . . . seen . . . my . . . uh . . . ?" she pleaded. "I have to . . . "

These children looked at me with compassionate, sad eyes which silently questioned as to how they should answer. "She's looking for someone who isn't here," I offered oddly, blinking to adjust my blurring vision. It was difficult to see her struggle.

Finally we arrived at the nurses' station. "Have you . . . seen . . . Norm?" She had not spoken her husband's name for a long time. The head nurse knew Norm and told Mom if she saw him she would let her know.

Once in her room she continued searching behind curtains and in the bathroom, all the while becoming more and more agitated. "I have to . . . I have to . . . " She dropped her head into her hands in a gesture of great sadness. And then came the full sentences: "I've . . . I've been gone so long. He's going to be so worried."

"Norm will come tomorrow. He isn't feeling well today." I was telling a partial truth. Norm was not well, though he didn't come to visit her even when he was well, and it was unlikely he would come tomorrow. This news about his well-being, however, intensified her sudden memory of her husband and her need to see him. Wringing her hands, then bringing her hands to her mouth, she inhaled deeply and released a sorrowful sigh. I didn't know what to do or how to help.

Mother was now frantic to return to her search, and she motioned for us to go. We returned to the hallway and continued to roam for what seemed to be a long time. I wondered about how she could manage to hold her determination to find Norm in her mind for such a long time. As we passed the nurses' station, I talked to a nurse about Mother's continued agitation. The nurse suggested that she take Mom to allow me to go home.

The next day the nurse said Mom's agitation had quickly subsided. I am not sure if that was the truth or if, instead, it was what I needed to hear.

CHAPTER 27

THE FEAR AND THE HOPE

Sorrow not, even as others who have no hope.
~ 1 THESSALONIANS 4:13

Mother lived a confused life for a long time. Once her decline became precipitous, news to the family was relayed fast and often. Her confusion increased; her appetite waned. She refused food entirely and then started eating again, just enough to keep herself going. Almost every month she lost weight, and every month she lost muscle strength. Her blood pressure was consistently low. She often had a low-grade fever. Soon she could barely stand and moved only with assistance.

Because she worked at the care facility, Lori had sat through hundreds of Wednesday care-plan meetings for her patients. Now it was her turn to attend the discussion of her mother's condition and hear the words, "Will your family want to consider hospice?"

Lori couldn't make that decision without us. All the children agreed hospice care was the next logical step. Though, logic had little to do with it, and "ready" wasn't the best descriptor of our consent. We all made plans to get home for the hospice meeting.

All the siblings arrived to find Mother drastically changed. More frail. Smaller. Her eyes focused within the room only when people arrived to call her back into the present. Then, she could rally and smile. But at times the gaze of her eyes seemed to focus in the distance. One time she pointed and then waved. She tried to speak to the distant point. And next she laughed.

I thought about the time our cousin Kay told us about her mom's last days. Aunt Wilma lived at home while Kay took care of her until the end when she was in hospice care. One morning Aunt Wilma told Kay that her Mama, her son, and her brother had been there to visit. Startled because these people had passed away long ago, Kay asked, "Well, what did they have to say?"

She answered, "Nothing. They were just sitting around living."

Aunt Wilma had become feisty and difficult as her body aged, but her memory was good. At the end, she went fast. For us, the loss of our mother happened over many years.

For so long we worried about Mother not knowing us, and then we worried about the agitation she must feel because she did not know us. This was the prevailing concern, right up to the day we listened to startling words she struggled to say. We knew she was trying to ask us something. When she found sounds to use, they came out as mumbles, but we could tell she was asking, "Who?" We were accustomed to pleas for help in finding the words that would tell her who we were and where she was and what all of us were doing there. I told her I was her daughter and waited to see if that helped.

But she stammered, her eyes intense. And then she finally managed, "Who . . . who am I?"

Our naive fear dissolved. Not knowing her children wasn't the most heartbreaking trouble Mother faced. With these words we knew she had lost her self. At times I had cried, fearing Mother would be gone when I arrived at the nursing home to visit her. This time I cried because she was still there. She was simply still there, lying in a bed doing nothing, being nothing. Alzheimer's disease took her from us while her physical body survived. She no longer knew who we were, and at this point she no longer knew who she was.

Lori and I stood by her bed, looking down at her and I blurted out, "I want her to go." I wanted her to get her wish for God to take her home and end this torturous journey. It would be easier. It would be better.

As the enormity of my thoughts weighed on my heart, Lori whispered, "I know. Me too."

I sobbed again when I told Regina about my dreadful thoughts. She shared that her friend had asked about whether we wanted to add Mother to the prayer chain. She told her friend no, although she did request her friend's personal and private prayers for Mom and for the family. But she couldn't ask people to pray that Mother would be spared from inevitable death or linger longer in a world she could not decipher. She certainly couldn't ask people to pray for Mother's quick death

We knew the day was coming and we feared the day was coming—that second loss—because we had lost her to the disease long before we lost her to death. It's incredibly difficult to watch your mother lose herself.

CHAPTER 28

HOSPICE

> Angels descending, bring from above,
> Echoes of mercy, whispers of love.
> ~ Fanny J. Crosby, "Blessed Assurance"

Oliver attended the meeting at which the family learned about hospice care. At only a month old, Oliver, Mother's youngest great-grandchild, slept soundly through the meeting to discuss the sudden downturn in Mother's health. All five of her children, our dad, and an adult granddaughter—Oliver's mother—were there, along with one teenage granddaughter and two pre-teen great-granddaughters, who sat respectfully for a while and then asked for money and took off for Starbucks. Oliver was healthy and content on his grandpa's chest. Somehow Oliver's presence seemed significant: a life ushered in and a life ushered out.

Hospice care provides support for terminally ill patients and their families. The care does not focus on curing the illness or prolonging life, nor does it hasten death. Instead it focuses on comfort and quality of life in the time that is left. Patients may be moved to hospice care when a doctor believes that the patient has a life expectancy of six months or less. Hospice care provides patients and families with a team of people—nurses and nurse's aides, social workers, counselors, chaplains, and volunteers. The team attends to medical needs, provides emotional support, and offers spiritual guidance.

People typically associate hospice care with patients who have terminal cancer or end-stage congestive heart failure. When doctors say that no additional treatments will change the outcome, hospice care helps patients have an alert, pain-free life in their last days, weeks, and months with a chance to live each day as fully as possible. A person like our mother who has Alzheimer's disease and is at the end of her expected lifespan presents a situation quite different from the situation of a cancer patient who has not reached expected time for end of life. Unlike a younger cancer patient, Mother could not tell anyone where it hurt, and she had lost quality of life long ago. Hospice care meets the individual needs of each kind of patient.

We had thought that hospice care was provided only in specific hospice facilities or in the home where a family member serves as the primary caregiver. Either of these circumstances is often the case. We learned, however, that hospice addresses people where they are—in hospitals, nursing homes, or assisted living facilities. Our meeting was with a hospice organization that worked with the nursing home where Mom resided. At that meeting we discussed Mother's move to hospice care within the nursing home. Our family agreed there would be no heroic scene of rushing her to the hospital to have an MRI or to address failing kidneys or to re-inflate a lung. The only heroic effort would be letting go of the hand that could still squeeze ours. The nursing facility would still be responsible for her care, hospice would be responsible for easing her comfortably through the end of life, and family members would still be her primary advocates.

As the hospice representative talked to us about the program, we learned that their consultation with Mom's doctor and their evaluation of her condition and medical records showed we had called them at the right time. She asked about the wishes of the family, and she asked many questions about Mother—who she had been and who she was now. Then, she outlined what would happen next.

The hospice staff started managing medication. No more medicines were given to treat the disease, nothing to keep her blood pressure under control or her cholesterol low. The nursing staff still dispensed medication, but it was the registered nurse from hospice who monitored it. The goal was palliative care—making her comfortable. After they were with Mom for a short time, the hospice staff could distinguish between confusion and pain. They treated the pain with morphine. When it wasn't enough, they gave more. No one worried about her becoming addicted. Mom received medicine to address stomach aches, bowel blockage, and hurts from falls, but nothing to fix her . . . nothing to prolong her life.

The hospice nurse said that Mother would tell us what she needed and how she was doing. She would not use words. We needed to stay tuned in to her non-verbal responses. If she refused food, it was because she did not need it to sustain her physical body for the next part of her journey. Activity level and appetite would fluctuate. Hospice staff would become her voice. They interpreted Mother's condition and needs for us, contacting the family often with personal phone calls and notes left in a journal for family members. They explained how they interacted with Mother at each visit.

Every day would be different, they said. In addition to the primary function of managing pain, they were there to manage practical details, address emotional challenges, and offer respite to the family. The family's job was to love her.

Patients often "perk up" when hospice arrives. People who are not old but face incurable illnesses sometimes feel better and live longer, especially if they enroll in hospice care early. Pain management is one reason people seem better. However, other services of the hospice team contribute significantly to patient improvement by managing depression and providing professional care.

After hospice care began for Mom, she seemed better too. She was getting more immediate attention from people who knew how to handle her and engaged with her in ways that returned her focus to the room she was in instead of the far off place to which she was traveling. Much of the temporary improvement came, however, because she no longer struggled with pain she could not communicate.

For patients who are not suffering from dementia, good hospice care sometimes forges strong relationships between the patient and the hospice staff. In Mom's case, hospice nurses grew attached to her, but there would be no meaningful relationship because she could no longer supply the effort to build her side of an alliance. They seemed to truly love Mom. Of course, the nursing home staff cared for her as well—but they were busy and had a whole wing full of patients who needed attention. The hospice nurse's aide and the volunteer were there as needed to comfort her by doing things such as feeding her, reading to her, and helping her dress.

Decisions about Mother's care were made according to a benefit vs. burden ratio: consideration of the benefit yielded by the care given when compared to the burden it added to the last days of her life. On certain days, getting Mother dressed burdened her in terms of pain and anxiety more than she benefitted from being dressed. Finding her frail body under the sheet dressed only in a diaper and brown socks distressed her daughters, but that didn't matter now. On bad days, being dressed wasn't worth the discomfort it caused.

A hospice social worker was there to address the family's emotional reactions. Patients who face death at a younger age than Mother benefit from a person trained to facilitate healthy social interactions. For so long we had worried about Mother's dwindling social contact, but at this point, when Mom communicated so little and so randomly, we realized the social worker was not there for Mom, but for us, the family. Information provided by hospice talked about families during times of stress. Often, families feel they are on an emotionally draining roller coaster ride. We were told to remember that the approaching death of a loved one rarely changes tangled and contentious family dynamics. Our family was grateful that our mother had raised children who got along. We had chosen to like each other as she had taught us.

As Mom lay there so fragile, so still, and so far away, she seldom spoke. One time when Lori leaned down to kiss her forehead as I straightened her bed, Mom took Lori's face, her hands cupping each cheek as she said, "I like you." Both of us felt the amazing and sustaining power of being liked—so much more purposeful than being loved, which is practically an obligation of motherhood. Being liked is a bonus because it's a choice.

We thought about stories of people who stay until a specific date or until all the children arrive or until some unfinished piece of business is concluded. The hospice nurse said the natural and expected rate of decline depends on the patient's non-cognitive drive. This non-cognitive drive—the will to live—is a curious thing. But how could that factor for a woman who had already lived past her sense of personhood? She was coasting on grace, physiologically present in her being. How does that line from "Amazing Grace" go? Mother would know it: "'T'is grace hath brought me safe thus far, and grace will lead me home."

For a little over three months Mother lingered with us. In the past I had often worried about the amount of time I had devoted to Mom. After she didn't know me specifically and after she first started introducing me as "one of her girls," she knew I was someone she was supposed to love if she could only figure out who I was. I took comfort in knowing my sisters were checking in with her. We were interchangeable parts. One day when I arrived to see Mom, the nurse's aide from hospice was feeding her. She talked about her fondness for Mom. She said Mom sometimes patted her knee and reached up to caress her cheek. These actions had been reserved for her daughters. Now the women on the hospice team were interchangeable parts as well.

As Mother worked harder and harder to breathe, our family discovered one unquestionable blessing of hospice care: the presence of nurses and social workers and chaplains and volunteers who understood exactly what was happening and knew what to expect. They knew what was normal, and this took away our fear of the unknown. We were in good hands. The situation was too big for us—for anyone—and we were freed to be small in the face of it, to be children of our mother. When the hospice nurse said, "You should spend as much time with your mom as you can today," I realized she had seen the signs and she knew.

Not long after, a commotion of text messages flew. Lori faced again a decision point that falls on the family member who is physically there. When do you start letting people know it looks bad and they better be ready?

Mother would be an atypical case of an elderly person who would die *from* Alzheimer's disease instead of *with* Alzheimer's disease. She had strong bones and a strong heart, both literally and figuratively, and she had no unfinished business.

CHAPTER 29

IT IS WELL WITH MY SOUL

> When peace like a river attendeth my way.
> When sorrows like sea billows roll;
> Whatever my lot, thou hast taught me
> to say, It is well, it well with my soul.
> ~ HORATIO GATES SPAFFORD, "IT
> IS WELL WITH MY SOUL"

Mother passed in the middle of the night when she and God decided she should be freed from the burden of Alzheimer's disease. Her daughter, Lori, was at her side. All her other children and her husband were on the way.

We have come to realize that our mother lived a good life—or, at the very least, she lived *her* life—rich with joys as well as sorrows. Her story need not be consumed by those last years as she struggled with the disease. The minister's funeral sermon recounted her admirable character, and the family in the pews bore witness to her life.

As well as looking back, a funeral looks forward without anyone being aware of it. A funeral looks forward when it is attended by little children wiggling in the pews, children who do not understand what has happened and sometimes need to be taken to the nursery, children like Audrey Elizabeth, who has her great-grandma's dimple in her right cheek, and who is not the last child born in a mother's line. That is the way of things.

Our mother's life will be measured by the children, grand-children, and great grandchildren who remain, like Abigail Mae who bears her name, and all the little ones to come, who will not know the grandmothers who came before them—Lilly Mae and Verna Mae and Jacque Mae.

So we forward-looking witnesses to our mother's life turn, as we always have, to what must be done. We gather up rambunctious children. We make sure the nursery is in order for the next little children who will use it. We thank the minister and ladies who served a meal. We make sure we have new phone numbers and email addresses of relatives we haven't seen for a while, and we go home. Mother goes home as well, to the life hereafter, as we have been taught, where we imagine her free of all ailments of body and mind. We leave the church secure in the joy that she is not lost without words in a scary world.

But we do not leave without learning that Avery and Arden continue to win golf tournaments . . . Max scored the winning goal at his soccer game and Noah scored the winning goal at hockey . . . Jeremy is visiting colleges . . . Taylor has mastered the backward flip . . . Cassidy is planning for law school . . . and Oliver is sleeping through the night. We go home to our lives, as Mother would have wanted.

This also is the way of things: these children and all the others will live lives rich with joys as well as sorrows and events their grandmothers never could have imagined. And they will have children who come into the world and go out of it in the usual way—without an instruction manual but with the promise of God's love.

POSTSCRIPT
WHAT CAN I DO TO AVOID MENTAL DECLINE?
(PLEASE DON'T SAY EXERCISE AND EAT RIGHT!)

> If I'd known I was going to live this long,
> I'd have taken better care of myself.
> ~ EUBIE BLAKE

PART 1

I looked it up. Apparently, the best strategy for staying both physically and mentally healthy well into old age is to exercise and eat right. Go figure! That, and having received a good genetic makeup at birth. Some things we can control and others we cannot.

First, let's discuss what we cannot control—specifically, the issue of Alzheimer's disease and heredity. The information presented here represents an examination of sources I judge to be reliable as a person who is not a scientist but is familiar with scholarly research. My goal is to present an easy-to-understand explanation of complex ideas.

In reporting research findings, scientists use language very precisely; they are not fond of generalization or distilling research to simplest explanations. Science is not so much a set of facts as it is a method of observation. When scientists state an observation, they pinpoint what has proved to be consistently true based on methodical and replicable examination. That's why translating it is so difficult for the rest of us . . . those of us who want an answer that we can easily understand but also count on to be true. Many things in life are not simple. Here's my best effort.

Alzheimer's disease is divided into two categories according to the age at which the disease is exhibited: early-onset AD occurring before age 65, and late-onset AD occurring after age 65. Some sources place the demarcation at 60, which tells us it's an arbitrary distinction. Of these two categories, late-onset AD is more prevalent.

As scientists continue work to discover why people get Alzheimer's disease, some of the focus is on the role of genetics in causing the disease. For some genetic disorders, the role that inherited genes play is pretty well understood. Examples of genetically inherited conditions include cystic fibrosis, sickle cell anemia, and color blindness. But with AD, the role of suspect genes in determining whether or not a child will also have the disease is less clear . . . well, murky . . . no, complicated. A survey of research suggests to me that three things are true: (1) for a narrow and specific subset of patients in the early-onset category, the genetic link to AD is confirmed; (2) for the majority of the patients in the early-onset category, there is no known connection between the genes of the patient and the disease; and (3) for the largest number of AD patients—those with late-onset Alzheimer's disease—the presence of a specific mutated gene is a risk factor for Alzheimer's disease, not a guarantee of its eventual manifestation.

Here's the explanation of statement #1. The condition of the small subset of patients in the early-onset category is called familial Alzheimer's disease (FAD). The National Institutes of Health considers early-onset familial Alzheimer's disease an inherited genetic disorder. That means they know this one is inherited—that this kind of AD runs in families because of the genetic information encoded in DNA. Scientists know that this kind of AD occurs as early as age 40, that it is rare, and that it is caused by the presence of at least one of three known gene mutations. When someone inherits one of these irregular genes, the result will (almost) always be Alzheimer's disease, generally at an early age. There is a 50/50 chance that a child will **not** inherit the mutated gene. However, inheriting the mutated gene will (almost) always result in manifestation of the disease (U.S. Department of Health, 2016).

While the inheritance factor for FAD is clear, the role of genetics in the rest of the early-onset category is unknown at this time (National Institute on Aging, 2016). As indicated in statement #2, researchers have not yet discovered the cause—or identified a connection to inherited genetic code—for the majority of cases of early-onset Alzheimer's disease.

Statement #3 refers to the other, larger category of Alzheimer's disease, patients with late-onset AD. For this group of patients, a specific mutated gene—but one different from the gene that causes familial AD—is the focus of research because it seems to be associated with the disease. The National Institute of Aging considers the presence of this gene a *genetic risk factor* for Alzheimer's disease, but not an inevitable cause of it (2016). The lack of clarity regarding a genetic connection for late-onset AD results because not everyone with the gene will get the disease. It's also true that not everyone who gets the disease will have the gene. More study of the disease will likely result in a clearer understanding of the connection between heredity and late-onset AD. But for now, late-onset AD is not labelled as an inherited genetic disorder. At present, the increased risk factor of developing late-onset AD when the person inherits the gene is only somewhat greater than the risk faced by the general population without the gene.

In other words, both types of AD have genetic components. However, late-onset AD is not considered a genetic disorder because the gene in question is not a consistent indicator of the likelihood of the disease. In addition, the disease may exist without the presence of the gene. The genes associated with FAD, on the other hand, consistently produce Alzheimer's disease. It's worth repeating that at the present state of research, the most consistently observed—the most reliable—risk factor for getting Alzheimer's disease is living to be old.

Since our mother suffered from late-onset Alzheimer's disease, this review of research provides good news for my siblings and me. Having a mother with the late-onset kind increases the risk for her children only slightly. None of us have decided to have the genetic testing that might provide clues about Alzheimer's disease before signs and symptoms appear. A blood test provides pieces of information about the presence or absence of genes associated with the disease, and as noted above, only for familial Alzheimer's disease does there appear to be a conclusive link. The test cannot predict the future for children with a parent who has late-onset AD. Too many other factors are involved . . . including lifestyle choices over which we have control.

PART 2

So let's talk about diet and exercise. Unlike the makeup of our genes, diet and exercise are factors we can do something about. The important connection between good nutrition and good health is hardly a news flash. "An apple a day keeps the doctor away," the old saying goes. Apparently, there's good reason to assume that apples protect against Alzheimer's disease. In addition to being beneficial in many other ways, apples provide a specific boost to the brain by increasing production of acetylcholine, a neurotransmitter, that helps the brain learn and form memories (Sauer, 2016). When apples facilitate production of acetylcholine, they are accomplishing one of the functions of some of the often prescribed AD drugs.

Unfortunately, we cannot say that if we merely drink two glasses of apple juice a day, we are good to go! There is no magic pill—or apple juice potion—that will cure or prevent AD. What we know for sure is that healthy diets help people become and stay healthy. Healthy foods containing vitamins and minerals protect against AD in the same way that all healthy foods, in adequate amounts and balanced supply, work to power the body and maintain healthy systems, whether it's good eye health, good heart health, or good brain health. There is some evidence about specific food positively affecting the health of the brain. But there is no research that says, "If you eat *this*, your brain will be healthy."

When we talk about diet, we need to stick to the evidence-based assumptions about specific foods and their relationship to good health. Reliable research shows that foods high in antioxidants may protect against AD (Davis, 2002). That means we should eat bright and colorful foods. Blueberries, blackberries, strawberries, asparagus, artichoke, and red cabbage are specifically touted. Drinking green tea is also recommended. Some studies have explored the possibility that coconut oil (organic, cold-pressed, non-hydrogenated, virgin coconut oil) can be beneficial as part of a brain-healthy diet (Napoletan, 2014).

A recent study revealed mice showed improvement in memory when fed a walnut-rich diet. Note that this study was partly funded by the California Walnut Commission (Sauer, 2014). Directing attention to that fact doesn't mean it's not true, but the sources of information should always be noted. The American Dairy Association (Fetters, 2014) has concluded from their studies that a few glasses of milk every day helps prevent Alzheimer's disease by raising the body's level of antioxidants. My search for information has revealed that any query that's titled "Can [insert current superfood here] prevent Alzheimer's disease?" is likely to arrive at an answer using the words, "Maybe" or "It's worth a try."

Other foods we are advised to include in our diets are those with vitamin E (nuts, seeds, fish oils, wheat germ), beta-carotene (liver, egg yolk, spinach, carrots, squash, broccoli, yams, tomatoes, cantaloupe, peaches, and grains), and also vitamin C (citrus fruits and juices and the colorful vegetables). Some sources suggest not peeling fruits and vegetables, apples and cucumbers specifically, because those brightest and most colorful parts contain the most nutrients. Some say that this advice counts only for organically grown produce. Any discussion seems to lead to additional paths to explore before we can be adequately informed about our food intake. There's a lot to learn. I once had a friend who told me she was so confused about diet, she had resorted to the simplest diet she could think of: If it tastes good, spit it out!

If we choose, however, to persevere on the subject, we learn that we should cut down on sweets, fats, and red meat. It's a good idea to have plenty of fish and fowl in our diets. Eat fish rich in Omega 3 fatty acids, specifically salmon, trout, and tuna. Some fat is required by the body. Moderate amounts of fats like those in milk and butter are actually good for us. Not so much if the three glasses are accompanied by a bag of Oreo cookies. The key word—just like the key word for most things in our lives—is "moderation."

We need to figure out which fats —in moderation—are the ones we need. Good fats are monounsaturated and polyunsaturated fats. Sources of good fats, in addition to those in fish, are nuts and vegetables like avocados; although, an avocado is technically a fruit.

The fats to stay away from are trans fats and saturated fats—and probably that container of bacon drippings Mom kept on the stove and dipped into generously when I was young. Trans fat is created in a lab, not by Mother Nature (except for tiny amounts naturally occurring in some meats and dairy products). The key phrase that indicates the presence of trans fat is "partially hydrogenated oils." The biggest purveyors of trans fats are processed foods: ready-made and packaged for sale.

Since the Food and Drug Administration determined in 2013 that trans fat is unsafe—reducing its intake could prevent thousands of heart attacks and deaths each year—more and more companies have voluntarily eliminated or reduced trans fats, including doughnut makers Krispy Kreme and Dunkin' Donuts. In fact, the FDA has required elimination of all trans fats in food products by 2018.

Elimination of trans fats doesn't mean some foods aren't loaded with calories from sugar and other fats, just that the calories are not the artery-clogging and laboratory-created trans fats. There will still be some trans fats in doughnuts and other products since they can round down to zero, and some trans fat is unavoidably produced during the manufacturing process.

Research has resulted in a good understanding of the diet needed for heart health. However, knowledge of what kind of diet may guard against AD is in early stages of investigation. At some future point, research may offer more conclusive information. One problem, of course, is that the study of memory, which is not an organ, is much more difficult than the study of the heart. Investigation thus far seems to suggest that the lists of beneficial foods may be the same for both heart and brain health. If it lowers cholesterol and is good for your heart, it's probably good for your brain. If it's not good for your heart, it's probably not good for your brain either.

Many doctors suggest checking out a Mediterranean diet, rich in fruits, vegetables, olive oil, legumes, whole grains, and fish because there is good evidence that foods included in this diet provide heart-healthy benefits. Now there are reasons to believe a Mediterranean diet may slow or reduce cognitive decline (Whiteman, 2016). Since people from India have a lower rate of AD than people from other regions of the world, researchers are interested in studying which elements of an Indian diet may protect against cognitive decline and how that protection may be happening in the brain. Ingredients of an Indian diet believed to support brain health include turmeric (the main ingredient in curry), ginger, and cinnamon.

So far, however, conclusive links between good brain health and the diet's role in sustaining it have proved elusive. Much more research is needed. We know for sure that nutrients (vitamins, minerals, carbohydrates, fats, proteins, and water) play important roles in good health. The discussion of how brain function is facilitated by these—as well as how that functioning is related to Alzheimer's disease—is long and complex. Many people turn to dietary supplements to get the nutrients believed to be important.

A wealth of information exists about what we should and should not eat and about which dietary supplements may or may not improve our diets. Not all of the info about diet and good brain health is easy to sort. We need vitamin E and choline and selenium and phosphatidylserine and potassium and magnesium and alpha-lipoic acid and niacin, etc., etc., etc. What is not complex and what engenders little disagreement is the idea that it's best to get the nutrition we need by eating real food. Food people eat . . . or used to eat before Doritos. All the nutrition we need is in a variety of . . . well, nutritious food—the fresher the better. But we at least need to consider the role of dietary supplements.

A dietary supplement is a product that contains one or more ingredients intended to add nutritional value to the diet. Determining if supplements will help us out is even more complicated than figuring out which "real" foods to eat. Although information abounds, not all information is created equal.

When scientists say they know something for sure, they always mean "for sure" within the limits of highly controlled investigation. In other words, they depend on empirical data. That's a good thing. When Aunt Betty swears by a brain-boost supplement, saying that it has really helped her to focus, she is offering anecdotal evidence, not empirical evidence. Good for Aunt

Betty—perhaps it's working for her, it probably isn't hurting her, and those dark chocolate bars she eats for aiding memory sure look yummy. But she is not offering proof based on evidence that extends beyond a sampling size of one person—Aunt Betty.

Sometimes anecdotal evidence—individual stories of effectiveness of a product reported by people like Aunt Betty—is the starting point for investigation using scientific methods. Such is the case with Ginkgo. Ginkgo, an herb which has been used as medicine for many years, is believed to be effective in addressing dementia and conditions associated with blood flow, as well as a list of disorders from asthma to hemorrhoids. Yet, the highest rating for efficacy that researchers gave Ginkgo is that it is "possibly effective" (Therapeutic Research Faculty, 2009). Ten other vitamins and supplements, among 54 substances studied, received this rating. None of the other 54 substances received a rating as hopeful as "possibly effective." The others were labelled "possibly ineffective" or "likely ineffective," with many drawing no conclusive finding because of insufficient evidence. (Findings were calculated using evidence-based reviews, without the influence of commercial interests, but were also based on user-generated reviews.) Just as no fountain of youth has been discovered to date, no magic substance has been discovered to cure or prevent Alzheimer's disease. Work continues to determine which foods and supplements contribute to brain health.

Dietary supplements believed to promote good brain health should not be considered equivalent to drugs approved to treat Alzheimer's disease. As mentioned in Chapter 10, Aricept, Razadyne, Exelon, Namenda, and Namzaric are the five drugs approved by the U.S. Food and Drug Administration (FDA) for marketing in the United States. Each claims to treat AD. Each drug was tested for safety and evaluated for effectiveness prior to being offered to the public. The FDA does not require that dietary supplements meet standards of pre-market regulation. Instead, supplements are regulated like food. Supplements have to be safe, in that they do not cause harm. Just as cantaloupe offered for sale to the public cannot have *Salmonella* in it, neither can supplements contain substances that endanger public health. The FDA withdraws from the market any supplements which prove to be harmful, but a drug cannot get to the marketplace *until* it is determined safe and also effective for the claim or claims that it makes.

If a dietary supplement claims to treat a disease, it must be regulated as a drug. A drug is defined by the FDA as a substance for which the intended use is the prevention, diagnosis, cure, mitigation, or treatment of a disease (U.S. Food and Drug, 2012). So if the manufacturer of a supplement claims that the product prevents, treats, or cures a disease, they are saying that it works like a drug, and the product must meet pre-market tests for safety and efficacy. For example, if a substance claims to treat arthritis, it must have the close scrutiny of pre-market approval. It's a drug. Arthritis is a disease, and any substance that treats it is, by definition, a drug. A dietary supplement cannot claim to treat arthritis, but a manufacturer may say that it "improves joint health."

Joint health is not a disease, so purporting the improvement of it does not fall within the definition for a drug. Remember, scientists act on what they know for sure. "Improvement" is subjective and hard to measure. Supplements offered to promote brain health are especially difficult to judge. Memory impairment is a much more complicated problem than, say, a problem with blood pressure. We know how to reliably calculate blood pressure and how to treat it with drugs that have been proved to work. It's hard to prove that a product doesn't work when no objective measurement is available.

The FDA does not interfere with commerce of manufacturers of supplements as long as their claims don't mark their products as drugs, which would initiate pre-market scrutiny, and as long as they don't say something that is verifiably untrue. There is always the chance that additional study—a different dosage, with a different population, in a different stage of a condition, or a host of other variables or narrowed range of factors—will prove the efficacy of a product by meeting the threshold of scientific proof.

As long as manufacturers of a product—or proponents of the program or remedy—say that it "may contribute" to a desired outcome or that "your results may vary," and as long as they do not make claims that define a substance as a drug, they are free to sell it and people are free to spend their money on whatever someone can convince them to buy.

Even when makers of dietary supplements, as well as a wide array of food products, meet standards of truthfulness, they may inadvertently—or purposefully—give information that misleads. Stating that a product is "all natural" is an example. "All natural" has no agreed upon meaning in the general population. Many consumers take the "all natural" label to mean that ingredients contained in the product are good for them. Yet just because something is "all natural" doesn't mean it won't harm users; just because something won't harm us doesn't mean it's good for us. Arsenic, anthrax, and hemlock are all natural, but each of them is dangerous if consumed. Even things that are beneficial can cause harm if not "taken as directed."

When thinking about improving health by supplementing our diets, there appears to be a very small category for "What We Know for Sure," while a large category exists for "What May Be True but There Is No Conclusive Data—Yet." When we move from the review of clinical trials, university studies, and respected laboratory research and into the world of commerce, we find a vast amount of information that fits in a category we might call "Not an Inkling of Evidence, but We'll Be Glad to Sell You Our Product."

So. What are we to do? We should choose foods that are believed to be healthy and won't do harm. If we decide to supplement food choices, we should choose ones that show *promise* of being effective. We should pay attention to the oft-repeated warning about consulting physicians before attempting uncontrolled treatment by any substance to account for dosage, length/method of use, and relationship to personal health factors. We should keep in mind the confines of trusted research—those clinical trials, university studies, and respected laboratory investigations. Research is necessarily limited in scope. When we assess claims people make about products or programs, the first question we should ask is, "Who says so?" The second question is, "What are their qualifications?" The third question, "Does the speaker profit from the information offered?"

Finally, we should learn that a single piece of information, a single kind of food, or a single vitamin supplement cannot solve the problems of health maintenance for our bodies. Even if we know for sure which foods or supplements work best to treat or postpone dementia and even if we avoid those foods that are *not good* for us and eat mostly foods that *are good* for us, we are not home free if we do not attend to lifestyle choices that impact our health.

PART 3

Exercise, for example, is important. We'd be hard pressed to find a doctor who denies the immediate and long-term health benefits of exercise for all patients in some individually appropriate amount.

Exercise makes people healthier. Exercise strengthens bones and muscles, and it reduces the risk of several diseases, including type 2 diabetes, cancer, cardiovascular disease, and various conditions associated with being overweight. Exercise can relieve stress, make people feel and look better, and give them more energy. Everyone knows this stuff already. Now the role of exercise in lowering the risk of cognitive decline has been explored.

Exercise not only improves blood flow to the brain, but recent studies also show that regular exercise produces chemicals that protect the brain. Improved memory, judgment, and thinking skills have been noted for people with mild cognitive impairment who regularly exercise, and studies show it slows the progress of AD (Mayo News Releases, 2013). More good news is that all the foods that are good for your brain are also good for maintaining an appropriate weight when eaten in appropriate quantities.

I chuckle when I hear television ads that say, "Lose 10 pounds for free!" Actually, you can lose all of the weight you want for free. Exercise is one-half of the formula for weight control, which is calculated by calories taken in versus calories burned. Burning off the calories consumed can be free or at least cheap. It just takes hard work.

I have a friend who battled with weight for a good part of her life. She accumulated the wreckage of a room full of exercise gadgets—everything from Thighmaster to stationary bikes to treadmills—and recalled a long list of broken New Year's resolutions. At last, while sweeping her arm Vanna White-style across the room, she said, "I can't buy another piece of equipment until someone invents something that will pick me up and throw me on one of these." Determination and willpower are hard to sustain. What helps many people is finding an exercise plan that fits them . . . and also setting attainable goals in small steps.

While it's true that physical exercise is good for brain health, it's also true that the brain itself needs exercise. People who stay active in mentally challenging activities are less likely to get AD (Speigel, 2014). Using your brain keeps it sharp because new nerve cells grow with mental stimulation and communication between those cells becomes stronger. Just as the brain needs exercise, it also needs to rest. People need downtime (Jabr, 2013).

Exercise for the brain needs to be something that represents a challenge to the brain. Once a person becomes skilled at a task, it's no longer new, and the brain doesn't have to work as hard. It becomes procedural memory. New challenges must be found or increased difficulty levels must be attempted. Consider engaged reading—especially reading aloud as it activates the use of additional brain cells. Intellectual discussion or any social engagement that requires interpreting and responding to information is good for the brain. We should tackle puzzles, card games, video games, or any game that requires strategy. Learning to play an instrument or learning a new language is good exercise for the brain. Even changing customary patterns of routine tasks is good exercise: driving home using a different route, brushing teeth with the non-dominant hand, folding clothes with eyes shut. Altering routine causes the brain to work harder. A brain working harder becomes stronger.

Because people with higher levels of education have a lower incidence of AD, lifelong learning should be a goal. Formal education may be protective because study requiring concentration and analytical thinking generate more brain cells with better connectivity. Having that good supply of brain cells in reserve may delay mental decline. But then, it could be that a high level of education generally leads to a less troubled life, one less impacted by bad health, more likely to afford a good diet . . . these factors also relate to lower incidence of AD or a delay in its symptoms. Vigorous engagement of the brain is not reserved for people who attend college or university.

My research has led me to discover that the scope of things we can do to prevent AD goes beyond diet and exercise to practically every facet of our lives. Getting enough sleep is crucial to good physical and brain health, as is staying hydrated and having friends. Things that are bad for the brain include smoking, heavy drinking, and stress. Preventing dementia—or at least keeping it at bay—may be dependent on making a hundred right choices. The problem is that we have to make those choices every single day.

Let's see if I can sort this out. The bottom line: we stay healthy if we do things that promote good health. Inversely, because having bad health leads to more bad health, we need to avoid behaviors—poor food choices as well as quality-of-life choices—that interfere with good health.

Our bodies are amazingly complex and extraordinarily balanced organisms, living in a world of highly complex social and environmental ecosystems. We do not live in some *Star Trek* version of the future when all diseases and their exact causes and precise cures have been figured out. We do not have a *Star Trek* sick bay with a Dr. McCoy who has a needle-less device that fixes us. We are still learning about our physical bodies, the least understood part of which is the brain and the central nervous system it controls. We are a long way from knowing everything we need to know. In the meantime, we can concentrate on doing the things that promote and sustain good health.

We will all be better off if we do the things we have always known to do. Eat healthy foods in moderation. Get enough sleep. Exercise both our bodies and our minds. Attend to our emotional well-being. And we might as well add love other people as much as we love ourselves. Sounds like a master plan that takes a lifetime. Just that easy; just that difficult. Thank you, Mom, for having taught me this all along.

DISCUSSION GUIDE FOR BOOK CLUBS

A variety of questions and quotes are presented for your consideration. Choose the ones that are most appropriate for your group. The quality of the discussion does not depend on the number of questions completed.

Good rules for good discussions: Everyone gets a turn to speak. Everyone's opinion is respected. Every contribution is valued.

I. FINISH THE SENTENCE

1. What I liked most about the book is . . .
2. What I liked least about the book is . . .
3. Most significant insight in the book . . .
4. What I would like to ask the author . . .
5. What I would like to know more about . . .
6. What I'm not sure I understand . . .
7. Most interesting idea or event described in the book . . .
8. Most surprising idea or event described in the book . . .
9. Most helpful fact included in the book . . .
10. Most helpful advice included in the book . . .

II. FOCUS ON A POINT.

1. The authors talk about losing their mother long before her death. When a loved one passes, most people experience five stages of grief: denial, anger, bargaining, depression and acceptance. Do you think the experience of losing someone to Alzheimer's disease follows the same

pattern? What do you think the author's might have learned about facing death?

2. Should people point out lapses in the memories of people with dementia? When they believe and repeat inaccurate information, is it best to correct them? Does it depend on what the information is? Does it depend on how the correcting is done?

3. Making a decision to care for a loved one at home or provide them with care in a nursing facility is a difficult one. Discuss.

4. In the chapter "What Role for the Fathers and Sons," the authors present the idea that women in the family shoulder the caregiving duties while men get a pass. Do you believe this is what happens most often in families or is it less frequent than the authors realize? If you are willing, share your experiences?

5. The authors' family had it easy compared to many people who care for a loved one at home. Some families deal with a loved one who is more aggressive or belligerent than their mother. Any thoughts? Do you think their attitudes in dealing with their mother would change had the circumstances been different?

6. Share your experiences of music eliciting memories of the past.

7. Do you agree that acceptance of a bad situation helps a person deal with the bad situation? Explain why or why not?

8. Discuss the need for caregivers to attend to their own health and emotional needs. How can caregivers address their own needs? How can others help? What are the support groups available to caregivers?

9. List strategies mentioned in the book, or other strategies you have discovered, for getting people with Alzheimer's disease or dementia to bathe. What about ways to get them to do other things you need them to do?

10. Discuss your thoughts on the current state of research on Alzheimer's disease. Consider the complexity of the brain. Consider the extent of the problem in a growing elderly population.

III. REACT TO A QUOTE

1. "We have come to realize that our mother lived a good life—or, at the very least, she lived *her* life—rich with joys as well as sorrows. Her story need not be consumed by those last years as she struggled with the disease." (Chapter 29)
2. "Whatever the circumstances that aided and abetted her loss of communication with friends, Mother was no longer experiencing social interaction that was challenging and reciprocal. I can now look back and see this time in her life as the beginning of the isolation that Alzheimer's disease imposes on its victims." (Chapter 6)
3. "Often memories are connected to music, and when songs of the time period are available to dementia patients, the music facilitates retrieval of information. They are able to recall who they were, where they were, and how they felt when they first heard Benny Goodman play 'In the Mood' or the time they sang along to Bing Crosby's 'I'll Be Seeing You.' For those not in my mother's generation, a different list of songs would retrieve memory." (Chapter 23)
4. "When prompting Mother to do something, we learned we should not explain why . . . when Mother's communication skills failed, talking about why an action was necessary became a waste of time for us and a source of frustration for her." (Chapter 25)
5. "When thinking about improving health by supplementing our diets, there appears to be a very small category

for 'What We Know for Sure,' while a large category exists for 'What May Be True but There Is No Conclusive Data—Yet.' When we move from the review of clinical trials, university studies, and respected laboratory research and into the world of commerce, we find a vast amount of information that fits in a category we might call 'Not an Inkling of Evidence, but We'll Be Glad to Sell You Our Product.'" (Postscript)

6. "She couldn't connect immediate circumstances to stories of the past. There could be no joke about her eating 87 pieces of broccoli, and she could not take solace in the knowledge of things having come full circle. You feed your daughter and then your daughter feeds you. She had lost so many things. I left Mother that day wishing she could understand that someone still cared if she ate her vegetables." (Chapter 16)

7. "We are sure it's true that families retell stories because shared experiences knit them together. Family stories chart their unique experiences . . . . These stories are shared joys and troubles we never tire of telling precisely because everyone knows how the story ends. It was easy to classify Mom's retelling of events as a part of this familial urge. Looking back, we know her stories were repeated not because we knew them well but because she thought we did not know them at all. The signs of Alzheimer's disease were right there for us to see." (Chapter 2)

8. "As he sat in his chair looking at the empty space where Mom's recliner had been, he said, 'I don't know how I let you kids talk me into this.' He said this without animosity. After he physically separated himself that day from his wife of almost 50 years, he occasionally—then seldom—visited her. The burden of his sadness was so great that he never went back to her emotionally." (Chapter 12)

9. "It must have been hard for her to have the thought right there on the tip of her tongue and yet be unable to communicate it. We learned to listen to what she meant, not what she said. We kept learning new things as Mom's condition worsened. I recall the time we learned that dementia patients may not remember new information . . . but they remember how they feel about it." (Chapter 25)

10. "As Mom lay there so fragile, so still, and so far away, she seldom spoke. One time when Lori leaned down to kiss her forehead as I straightened her bed, Mom took Lori's face, her hands cupping each cheek as she said, 'I like you.' Both of us felt the amazing and sustaining power of being liked—so much more purposeful than being loved, which is practically an obligation of motherhood. Being liked is a bonus because it's a choice." (Chapter 28)

IV. IF YOU ARE WILLING, SHARE A PERSONAL EXPERIENCE OR YOUR FAMILY'S EXPERIENCE WITH ALZHEIMER'S DISEASE OR SOME OTHER FORM OF DEMENTIA.

REFERENCES

ABC News. (2014, March 5). iPods Awaken Memories Through Music for Those With Alzheimer's. Retrieved from World News, http://abcnews.go.com/blogs/health/2014/03/05/ ipods-awaken-memories-through-music-for-those-with-alzheimers/.

Alzheimer's Association. (2016a). Alzheimer's Myths. Retrieved from http://www.alz.org/alzheimers_disease_myths_about_ alzheimers.asp.

Alzheimer's Association. (2016b) Medications for Memory Loss. Retrieved from http://www.alz.org/alzheimers_disease_myths_about_alzheimers.asp.

Alzheimer's Association. (2016c). Latest Facts and Figures. Retrieved from http://www.alz.org/facts/.

Ashford, M. (2010, August 31). How Are Memories Stored in the Brain? Retrieved from LiveScience, http://www.livescience. com/32798-how-are-memories-stored-in-the-brain.html.

Bergland, Christopher. (2013, December 11). Why Do the Songs from Your Past Evoke Such Vivid Memories? *Psychology Today*. Retrieved from https://www.psychology today.com/blog/the-athletes-way/201312/why-do-the-songs-your-past-evoke-such-vivid-memories.

Clair, A. (2016, January 28). Education and Care: Music. Retrieved from Alzheimer's Foundation of America, http://www. alzfdn.org/EducationandCare/musictherapy.html.

Darabont, F. (Director) & Darabont, F. (Writer). (1994). *The Shawshank Redemption* [Motion picture]. United States: Columbia Pictures.

Davis, J. (2002, June 25). Antioxidants Fight Alzheimer's. Retrieved from WebMD News Archive, http://www.webmd.com/alzheimers/news/20020625/antioxidants-fight-alzheimers.

Fetters, K. (2015, April 17). Can Drinking Milk Prevent Alzheimer's Disease? *U.S. News & World Report.* Retrieved from http://health.usnews.com/health-news/health-wellness/articles/2015/04/17/can-drinking-milk-prevent-alzheimers-disease

Golby A., Silverberg, G., Race, E., Gabrieli, S., O'Shea, J., Knierim, K., Stebbins, G., Gabrieli, J. (2005, February 10). Memory encoding in Alzheimer's disease: an fMRI study of explicit and implicit memory. Brain: A Journal of Neuroscience, 128(4), 773-789; http://dx.doi.org/10.1093/brain/awh.

Hsu, J. (2009, February 24). Music-Memory Connection Found in Brain. Retrieved from *LiveScience,* http://www.livescience.com/5327-music-memory-connection-brain.html.

Huppert, B. (2014, December 8). Choir of Alzheimer's patients sings tunes from memory. *USA Today.* Retrieved from https://www.usatoday.com/story/news/nation-now/2014/12/08/inspiration-nation-alzheimer-choir/19964747/.

Jabr, F. (2013, October 15). Why Your Brain Needs More Downtime. *Scientific American.* Retrieved from https://www.scientificamerican.com/article/mental-downtime.

Lerner. M. (2016, October 11). Alzheimer's researchers at University of Minnesota reverse memory loss in mice. *Star Tribune.* Retrieved from as http://www.startribune.com/alzheimer-s-researchers-at-university-of-minnesota-reverse-memory-loss-in-mice/396739231/.

Lieff, J. (2015, December 23). The Role of Tau in Brain Function and Dementia. Retrieved from Searching for the Mind, http://jonlieffmd.com/blog/human-brain/the-role-of-tau-in-brain-function-and-dementia.

Mastin, L. (2010a). Declarative (Explicit) & Procedural (Implicit) Memory. Retrieved from The Human Memory, http://www.human-memory.net/types_declarative.html.

Mastin, L. (2010b). Episodic & Semantic Memory. Retrieved from The Human Memory, http://www.human-memory.net/types_episodic.html.

Mayo Clinic Staff. (2016). Alzheimer's Treatments: What's on the Horizon? Retrieved from Mayo Clinic, http://www.mayoclinic.org/diseases-conditions/alzheimers-disease/in-depth/alzheimers-treatments/art-20047780.

Mayo News Releases. (2013, January 25). Exercise Best Medicine to Prevent Alzheimer's. Retrieved from Mayo Clinic News Network, http://newsnetwork.mayoclinic.org/discussion/exercise-best-medicine-to-prevent-alzheimers/.

Napoletan, A. (2014, August 20). Can Coconut Oil Prevent Alzheimer's? Retrieved from Alzheimers.net, http://www.alzheimers.net/2013-05-29/coconut-oil-for-alzheimers/.

National Institute of Neurological Disorders and Stroke. (2015, November 2). Dementia: Hope Through Research. Retrieved from National Institutes of Health, www.ninds. nih.gov/disorders/dementias/detail_dementia.htm.

National Institute on Aging. (2015, January 22). Alzheimer's Disease: Unraveling the Mystery: The Hallmarks of AD. Retrieved from National Institutes of Health, https://www. nia.nih.gov/alzheimers/publication/part-2-what-happens-brain-ad/hallmarks-ad.

National Institute on Aging. (2016, September 29). Alzheimer's Disease Genetics Fact Sheet. Retrieved from Alzheimer's Disease Education & Referral Center, the National Institutes of Health, https://www.nia.nih.gov/alzheimers/publication/alzheimers-disease-genetics-fact-sheet#alzheimers.

Norton, A. (2015, May 19). Alzheimer's-Tied Brain Plaque May Precede Symptoms. Retrieved from WebMD News Archive, http://www.webmd.com/alzheimers/news/20150519/alzheimers-linked-brain-plaques-may-arise-decades-before-symptoms.

PubMed Health. (2016, March 17). Memories "taken" by Alzheimer's could possibly be retrieved. Retrieved from U.S. National Library of Medicine, http://www.ncbi.nlm.nih.gov/pubmed-health/behindtheheadlines/news/2016-03-17-memories-taken-by-alzheimers-could-possibly-be-retrieved/.

Punsky, K. (2015, March 23). Mayo Clinic Study of Thousands of Brains Reveals Tau as Driver of Alzheimer's Disease. Retrieved from Mayo Clinic News Network, http://news-network.mayoclinic.org/discussion/mayo-clinic-study-of-thousands-of-brains-reveals-tau-as-driver-of-alzheimers-disease/.

Reid, T. (2015, January/February). When Will the War on Alzheimer's Begin? *AARP Bulletin. 56(1)* 15–20.

Sample, I. (2013, November 11). Alzheimer's patients' brains boosted by belting out Sound of Music. Retrieved from *The Guardian,* https://www.theguardian.com/science/2013/nov/11/alzheimers-patients-brains-boosted-sound-music-singing.

Sauer, A. (2014, October 24). Eat Brain-Boosting Walnuts to Prevent Alzheimer's. Retrieved from Alzheimers.net, http://www.alzheimers.net/10-24-14-walnuts-prevents-alzheimers.

Sauer, A. (2015, February 5). Apple Juice May Help with Brain Cognition. Retrieved from Alzheimers.net, http://www.alzheimers.net/2-5-15-apple-juice-alzheimers-prevention/.

Schaeffer, J. (2016, September/October). Music Therapy in Dementia Treatment—Recollection Through Sound. *Today's Geriatric Medicine.* Retrieved from http://www.todaysgeriatricmedicine.com/news/story1.shtml.

Scuitt, S. (2016, September). Is new Alzheimer's drug a game-changer? Retrieved from CNN, http://www.cnn.com/2016/08/31/health/experimental-alzheimers-drug/).

Speigel, B. (2014, February 18). 5 Ways to Fight Dementia Daily: Learn Something New Today. Retrieved from Everyday Health, http://www.everydayhealth.com/alzheimers-pictures/daily-to-dos-to-combat-dementia-risk.aspx#04.

Suomen Akatemia (Academy of Finland). (2011, December 6). Listening to Music Lights Up the Whole Brain. *ScienceDaily*. Retrieved from www.sciencedaily.com/releases/2011/12/111205081731.htm.

Therapeutic Research Faculty. (2009). Common Vitamins and Supplements Used to Treat Alzheimer's Disease. *WebMD*. Retrieved October 7, 2016, from Natural Medicines Comprehensive Database Consumer Version, http://www.webmd.com/vitamins-supplements/condition-981-Alzheimer's+disease.aspx?print=true.

U.S. Department of Health and Human Services. (2016, October 4). Alzheimer's disease: Inheritance pattern. Retrieved from Genetics Home Reference, U.S. National Library of Medicine, National Institutes of Health, https://ghr.nlm.nih.gov/condition/alzheimer-disease#sourcesforpage.

U.S. Food and Drug Administration. (2012, February 2). Drugs@FDA Glossary of Terms. Retrieved from Drug Approvals and Databases, http://www.fda.gov/Drugs/InformationOnDrugs/ucm079436.htm.

Whiteman, H. (2016, August 10). Mediterranean diet may slow cognitive decline, prevent Alzheimer's. *Medical News Today*. Retrieved from http://www.medicalnewstoday.com/articles/312246.php.

World Health Organization. (2015, March). Dementia Fact Sheet. Retrieved from http://www.who.int/mediacentre/factsheets/fs362/en/.

ACKNOWLEDGEMENTS

We are forever grateful to our husbands, Ron and John, who have been patient and kind during the writing of this book. We also thank Grace Eckland and members of the Lake Havasu City Writers Group.